"Absolutely brilliant! A must-read for all Amer... tial yet practical guide to solving your pain problems."

– Robin Raju, DO, assistant professor,
orthopaedics and rehabilitation, Yale School of Medicine

"A remarkable book, full of empathy and empowerment for those suffering from chronic pain. Dr. Sharma's Relief-5R plan informs and supports us to make clear and reachable steps to markedly reduce pain and enhance health!"

– Erik Ensrud, MD, professor of physiatry and neurology, University of Kansas

"Dr. Sharma's book empowers the patient, illuminates nondrug remedies, and revives practitioners' treatment repertoires. It is a great resource for those confronting pain."

– Ronnen Abramov, DO, pain medicine specialist, Princeton Medical Center

"This book is a critical read for anyone suffering from chronic pain and in need of tangible, concrete strategies to get back to a more normal life, one less reliant on medications and instead more focused on centering activities that improve overall wellness. It's so timely, given the havoc the Covid-19 pandemic has wreaked on many individuals suffering with chronic pain and addiction disorders."

– Vin Gupta, MD, MPA, professor and health policy expert; senior principal, health, at Amazon; and medical analyst at NBC News

"Dr. Saloni Sharma's book provides empathic, sound clinical advice to the millions of patients experiencing and managing chronic back pain. Dr. Sharma's Relief-5R plan is a helpful approach that enables patients to set small goals toward creating lasting habits. I love how she describes them as 'microboosts' — 'little steps that boost you toward ease and relief.' I know my patients will benefit from Dr. Sharma's guidance and techniques."

– Deborah A. Venesy, MD, senior staff, Cleveland Clinic Center for Spine Health

"*The Pain Solution* offers what the title promises. You can, by reading this book, discover your best self and be free of the pains of your past. Read, learn, and be guided to a more comfortable life, and let the healing begin!"

– Bernie Siegel, MD, *New York Times* bestselling author of *Love, Medicine & Miracles* and *No Endings, Only Beginnings*

"Dr. Sharma offers a simple framework and reasonable strategies to navigate an often complicated and daunting path to optimal health. I will wholeheartedly recommend this book to my patients, friends, and family."
— **John Vasudevan, MD, CAQSM,** associate professor, University of Pennsylvania, and medical director, Rock 'n' Roll Philadelphia Half Marathon

"Chronic pain is arguably the most soul-sapping, joy-gutting adversity an ever-increasing portion of our population — our loved ones, colleagues, selves — struggles with every day. Dr. Sharma's groundbreaking and scientifically solid book upshifts us from victims to healers. *The Pain Solution* equips us with a potent and vital blend of self-efficacy, action, hope, and control. This is the book you will want to give to anyone and everyone who is in pain and suffering."
— **Paul G. Stoltz, PhD,** globally bestselling author of *Adversity Quotient* and *GRIT* and founder and CEO of PEAK Learning, Inc.

"Dr. Sharma has outlined a tremendous process that will help all people who suffer from chronic pain. Her five-step solution applies to anyone with any type of chronic pain and is a great series of options that patients can use in the comfort of their own homes to relieve (or prevent the occurrence of) pain. Dr. Sharma is an incredible colleague who is world-renowned for her conservative and effective treatment options for patients with chronic pain, and it is no surprise that she has written a seminal work on this topic."
— **Ameet Nagpal, MD, MS, MEd,** division chief, physical medicine and rehabilitation, Medical University of South Carolina

"As a physician who sees patients in pain on a daily basis, Dr. Sharma has written a must-read book for all who have ever had debilitating pain to learn how to regain control of their lives and pursue the version of themselves they can only dream of now. This is the most comprehensive but approachable guide to why we hurt and what we can do about it. It starts with a self-assessment that allows us to identify opportunities for growth and improvement, then shows us how to achieve them. For those of us currently hurting, she helps us understand how we got to where we are — and how to get out of there!"
— **Ai Mukai, MD,** faculty, Dell Medical School, University of Texas at Austin, and pain management specialist, Texas Orthopedics Sports and Rehabilitation, OrthoLoneStar, Austin

The Pain Solution

The Pain Solution

5 Steps to Relieve and Prevent Back Pain, Muscle Pain, and Joint Pain without Medication

Saloni Sharma, MD, FAAPMR, LAc

Foreword by Andrew Weil, MD

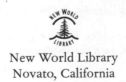

New World Library
Novato, California

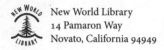 New World Library
14 Pamaron Way
Novato, California 94949

Text design by Tona Pearce Myers

Library of Congress Cataloging-in-Publication Data

Names: Sharma, Saloni, author.
Title: The pain solution : 5 steps to relieve and prevent back pain, muscle pain, and joint
    pain without medication / Saloni Sharma, MD, FAAPMR, LAc ; foreword by Andrew
    Weil, MD.
Description: Novato, California : New World Library, [2022] | Includes bibliographical
    references and index. | Summary: "A patient-proven approach to pain prevention,
    relief, and eradication without medication, surgery, or special equipment"--
    Provided by publisher.
Identifiers: LCCN 2022000218 (print) | LCCN 2022000219 (ebook) | ISBN
    9781608687930 (paperback) | ISBN 9781608687947 (epub)
Subjects: LCSH: Pain--Alternative treatment. | Backache--Alternative treatment. |
    Myalgia--Alternative treatment. | Joints--Diseases--Alternative treatment.
Classification: LCC RB127 .S46 2022 (print) | LCC RB127 (ebook) | DDC
    616/.0472--dc23/eng/20220126
LC record available at https://lccn.loc.gov/2022000218
LC ebook record available at https://lccn.loc.gov/2022000219

First printing, May 2022
ISBN 978-1-60868-793-0
Ebook ISBN 978-1-60868-794-7
Printed in Canada on 100% postconsumer-waste recycled paper

 New World Library is proud to be a Gold Certified Environmentally Responsible Publisher. Publisher certification awarded by Green Press Initiative.

10   9   8   7   6   5   4   3   2   1

To all the people searching for relief, ease, and joy

To all the patients I have had the honor of treating

To my colleagues making a difference in a fractured system

And to my loves, for their unwavering support, love, and belief:
MW, LW, MW, Dad, Mom, MS, and PS

A bird slams into the glass.
A bird slams into the glass.
A bird slams into the glass.
Over and over again, headfirst,
determined to defeat its own reflection.
A head butt of bravado.
I watched it, time and time again.
From the inside, I studied the dozens of oily streaks
smeared across the window.
After a few minutes, the bird would fly away — sore or distracted
from its battle with itself.
It would be comical if it weren't painful.

Like the bird, we repeatedly bash ourselves against
invisible constraints:
eat poorly, sleep less, move less, enjoy less human connection,
take on more responsibilities, build stress, and suffer more.

It is time to stop beating ourselves against the glass.
To pause and to be mindful.
To see who we are.
To decide who we are becoming,
what our body is becoming,
and what our life is becoming.
Let's stop ramming into the glass.
Let's stop suffering.
Let's ease pain.
Let's live better.

SALONI SHARMA, MD

Contents

Foreword

We have a big problem. More people are suffering from pain than ever before — with devastating consequences. More than one in every five Americans report ongoing pain, especially back, joint, and muscle pain. For decades the pharmaceutical industry has pushed medications as the primary treatment for pain — anti-inflammatories, muscle relaxers, and dangerous opioids. These medications are not solutions, merely ways to temporarily dampen symptoms. Worse, they often have adverse effects and such unintended consequences as organ damage, bleeding ulcers, brain fogginess, constipation, breathing abnormalities, addiction, and even death. The painful conditions they are used for would be better treated by improving eating patterns, activity levels, sleep habits, and stress levels. A true pain solution must go to the source of the problem and address the whole person. This book offers a true pain solution. As you read it, you will discover that lasting pain relief is not found in pill bottles but rests on building a healthy lifestyle, pain resiliency, and preventative measures. It is time to take charge of our own pain care. It is time to stop suffering.

Although the United States is a beacon of scientific achievement and medical innovation, compared to other nations it has one of the highest rates of people in pain. Low back pain is the number one cause of disability in our country. Because of our nation's pharmaceutical-driven medical approach, we lead the world in opioid use and are fighting an opioid crisis. Unfortunately, physicians in training are not typically taught other ways to treat pain, and many patients are not aware of evidence-based, nonpharmacological treatments.

In my role as director of the Andrew Weil University of Arizona Center for Integrative Medicine, I have taught thousands of physicians, allied health professionals, and students about other ways to treat pain. One example is dietary change. When I develop a treatment program for a patient, my first step considers ways to change eating patterns that can help. An anti-inflammatory eating plan can calm pain. There is excellent evidence that supports this, and Dr. Sharma skillfully explains the data while providing practical recommendations on how to take advantage of it. Another possibility is mind-body medicine, making use of mindfulness, meditation, breathing exercises, guided imagery, and visualization. Patients often experience remarkable pain relief with these methods. This book not only reveals the evidence behind these methods but shares a novel approach for comprehensive pain relief.

Dr. Sharma is a double board-certified pain physician, a national leader in pain management, medical director of the Orthopaedic Integrative Health Center, an acupuncturist, and a graduate fellow in integrative medicine at the University of Arizona. This book is a culmination of her years of work managing orthopaedic pain with both conventional and integrative treatments. *The Pain Solution* fills an urgent need. It is what we have been searching for to understand and implement better pain care. This is the future of medicine — treating the whole person, not just the symptom. In this integrative approach, we all play an active role in our care, build wellness, improve resiliency, and live better.

Congratulations on starting the journey to a better life with less pain!

ANDREW WEIL, MD
Tucson, Arizona

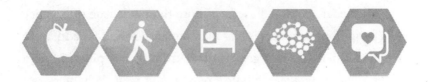

Introduction

Two metal rods ran the length of my spine. A third metal rod emerged from the plastic that encased my abdomen, lay across my breastbone, and met the other rods to form a ring around my neck like a metal dog collar. Little screws on the back of the brace tore out strands of my hair. I was eleven years old, and this was the treatment for a curved spine. From this experience, I learned what it meant to live with orthopaedic pain long before I became a physician certified in treating people with pain. Experiencing orthopaedic pain inspired my mission to help people live better and with less pain.

Fortunately, most people do not spend years encased in metal restraints, but an estimated 80 percent of Americans experience back pain at some point in their lives. This statistic does not take into account other types of orthopaedic pain, including muscle sprains, arthritis pain, joint pain, and neck pain. While orthopaedic pain may seem inevitable for most people, we can lessen its impact on our daily lives. We can reduce its intensity and duration, protect ourselves against future pain, and stop suffering by making small changes in the way we live. These small steps move us toward ease and relief. I call them *microboosts*.

My Relief-5R plan, based on more than a decade of practice as a pain physician, consists of many microboosts that add up to big pain relief. The plan gets its name from its five pillars of pain relief: *refuel, revitalize, recharge, refresh, and relate*. Chapters 3–7 of the book discuss each of these pillars in depth and offer a wide range of microboosts that have proved effective in reducing and preventing pain. Level 1 microboosts are small, simple changes that you can implement right away; level 2 microboosts may require a little more time, effort, or commitment. To help these microboosts stick, each chapter contains practical advice for easily integrating them into your routine. This is the road map to less pain, more function, and a better life.

Does pain limit you now? Do you want to prevent pain from hijacking your life? The questionnaire below identifies key risk factors for chronic pain and suffering. Thankfully, we can eliminate most of these risk factors and reduce others; only a few are part of our history. And even though we cannot change that history, we can change our view of it so that we are not shackled by pain.

It may be helpful to complete this questionnaire once before you begin the Relief-5R plan and again after you have followed it for four weeks. This is a living experiment: test out the plan and see if it works for you. After all, you have nothing to lose but pain and suffering.

Risk Factors for Chronic Pain: Questionnaire

Respond to these questions on a scale from 0 to 5, where 0 means "no" or "never," and 5 means "yes" or "always."

1. Do you have recurring pain?

0   1   2   3   4   5

2. Are you overweight?

0   1   2   3   4   5

3. Do you eat processed foods and sugary foods more than twice a day? (This includes packaged foods with more than five ingredients and foods with more than ten grams of added sugar.)

0   1   2   3   4   5

4. Do you have a low intake of vegetables, fruits, nuts, and fish?

0   1   2   3   4   5

5. Do you consume sugary beverages, including soda, fruit juice, or coffee or tea with sugar daily ?

0   1   2   3   4   5

6. Do you drink less than four glasses of water a day?

0   1   2   3   4   5

7. Are you sedentary for most of the day?

0   1   2   3   4   5

8. Do you walk for less than twenty minutes a day?

0   1   2   3   4   5

9. Do you take anti-inflammatory medications (e.g., ibuprofen, naproxen) daily or nearly every day?

0   1   2   3   4   5

10. Do you smoke?

0   1   2   3   4   5

11. Do you drink alcohol daily?

0   1   2   3   4   5

12. Do you spend limited time outside daily?

0   1   2   3   4   5

13. Do you sleep for less than seven hours a night?

0   1   2   3   4   5

14. Do you have trouble sleeping?

0   1   2   3   4   5

15. Do you have any inflammatory conditions, such as diabetes, prediabetes, heart disease, or high blood pressure?

0   1   2   3   4   5

16. Do you have family members with chronic pain?

0   1   2   3   4   5

17. Do you have a history of adverse childhood experiences (trauma, abuse, neglect)?

0   1   2   3   4   5

18. Do you have trouble coping with change?

0   1   2   3   4   5

19. Are you under stress?

0   1   2   3   4   5

20. Do you find it difficult to deal with stress?

0   1   2   3   4   5

21. Are you no longer learning something new or challenging yourself?

0   1   2   3   4   5

22. Do you feel lonely?

0   1   2   3   4   5

23. Are you surrounded by negative people who bring you down?

0   1   2   3   4   5

24. Do you have a pessimistic outlook?

0   1   2   3   4   5

25. Do you have days when you experience no joy?

0   1   2   3   4   5

Add up your numerical responses to all the questions. If your score is higher than 30, then you may have a higher risk of chronic pain and suffering. The good news is that many of these factors can be modified with little tweaks to your daily routine. The Relief-5R plan provides simple steps to reduce and prevent pain. The following pages will explain how to put it into practice. As with all health and wellness changes, please clear all changes with your own physician before you begin.

❖

Congratulations on starting a path to a better life!

CHAPTER 1

The Pain Problem

The way modern medicine operates is like trying to diagnose what's wrong with your car by listening to the noises it makes instead of looking under the hood....
We must learn to treat the person, not the disease; the system, not just the symptoms.

— MARK HYMAN, MD

If you are the kind of person who believes in treating the root cause of pain instead of relying on temporary Band-aids, then this is the book for you. We can calm pain, build resilience, and stop suffering without medications. True relief comes from identifying and treating the source of pain. Think about the last time you felt good, living your life with joy and without pain, your body well, and your mind calm. Can you see it? Can you feel it? It is possible to feel that way again. We can design our lives to help us feel better, be better, and live better.

You may want to prevent severe pain, or you may have struggled with crippling pain for days, months, or years, with little relief provided by conventional remedies. But painful suffering is not your destiny. Failed treatments are not your fault. There is a lot of misinformation and impractical advice out there, often spread by those with ulterior motives. Continued pain, information overload, and a pain-induced brain fog may conspire to prevent us from feeling better.

For more than a decade I have helped people who were suffering with excruciating back, neck, muscle, and joint pain. The best outcomes occur when we treat the cause of the pain rather than the symptom of pain. A few years ago, Cindy, a 45-year-old woman, came to see me after battling chronic back pain with unpredictable, debilitating pain flares for over two decades. She had tried anti-inflammatories, muscle relaxers, and pain pills. At times, these gave her temporary, slight relief but always left her with side effects, from heartburn and constipation to daytime sleepiness. On some days she could not even get dressed by herself because of the pain. Cindy lived in fear of her back "going out." She continued to work and to care for her loved ones, but she stopped caring for herself. To try to avoid pain flares, she stopped exercising, hiking with her friends, and doing other fun activities. The pain seeped into every aspect of her life. Cindy lived in fear — isolated, inactive, and unhappy. Slowly she put on weight, and this worsened not only her pain but also her diabetes, high blood pressure, and depression. While she was able to manage the dull, constant pain, the seemingly unpredictable, severe flares brought her to her knees several times a year. She was tired of ineffective medications with troublesome side effects. Cindy wanted to feel better and live better.

We developed a plan based on my Relief-5R program to reduce her pain and inflammation. Within fourteen days of starting the plan, she was more active and felt less stressed. She started eating healthier food, taking short hikes with her friends, and sleeping better. After three months, she had not had a single painful flare-up.

Her daily pain was now mild. After six months, she had a back flare after helping a friend move into an apartment, but it lasted only one day, and she recovered easily. The severe attacks of pain are gone. Cindy now lives free of debilitating pain, fear, and suffering.

In this book, we address the root causes of pain and inflammation and the factors that aggravate them, and we will develop a plan that will enable you, like Cindy, to live fully with less pain and fewer medications.

If pain has prevented you from doing something you enjoy, picture yourself doing that activity with ease, without potentially dangerous medications and free of the fear of a painful flare. If you have been a hostage to pain, you can free yourself and live a whole, balanced life again with the Relief-5R plan.

Pain in the USA

In a one-year period, more than 54 percent of Americans report musculoskeletal pain, including arthritis pain, low back pain, and neck pain. The search for relief has created a different kind of epidemic. The opioids frequently prescribed for pain relief have created a crisis of addiction, shattering families and stealing more than forty-five thousand lives a year. Other pain medications, like nonsteroidal-anti-inflammatory medications (NSAIDs), damage our internal organs and claim more than ten thousand lives a year. We turn to these medications because we are offered no other path to pain relief or prevention. We have a medication crisis because we have a pain crisis. Pain hijacks lives, destroys families, and disables communities.

Severe pain limits routine activities like getting dressed and walking. It keeps us from fully participating in life. Low back pain alone causes more disability than any other medical condition in the United States and worldwide. In the United States, musculoskeletal disorders and neck pain are the third and fourth leading causes of disability, and arthritis ranks in the top ten. Of the top four causes of disability, three of them are spine and musculoskeletal issues. Often, the second leading cause, depression, is linked to ongoing pain. Incapacitating pain prevents caring for ourselves, caring for loved ones, and enjoying a good quality of life. Pain riddles our country, and the number of people hampered by chronic pain keeps increasing.

We may have heard of nonpharmacological ways to treat pain or reduce inflammation, but these approaches are not advertised with Super Bowl commercials or full magazine spreads. Improving our food intake, sleep, movement, and stress levels are measures that don't help sell pills or food products. Massive industries spend billions of dollars a year to keep us misinformed and dependent on their products. For example, the processed food industry orchestrates our addiction to nutrient-poor, processed foods loaded with inflammatory sugars, salts, carbohydrates, and fats. These foods make us feel worse but keep us coming back for more. Similarly, big pharmaceutical companies want you to believe that you need addictive, expensive, and potentially deadly medications to feel better. They are wrong.

Without being offered viable alternatives to medication, many of us are left trapped in pain. Experiencing chronic pain is not the result of mistakes, indifference, laziness, or lack of willpower to eat healthy foods or exercise more. But neither is it an unalterable destiny. My Relief-5R plan is based on making small personalized tweaks to diet, movement, stress levels, mindset, and environment that help us to function better and live every day with less pain, less inflammation, and less disability.

Some people fear that making choices that promote wellness will require time-consuming, disruptive, or expensive changes to their lives, but the Relief-5R plan makes it easy: you choose the changes that will work for you. In addition, it offers huge potential gains. Do you have more energy after you eat real, unprocessed food? Do you feel better when you do some type of self-paced movement? Does your day go more smoothly if you have had enough sleep? Do you handle stress better when you take just ten minutes to reset? Do you feel happier when you spend time with people you care about? The answer to these questions is usually yes — or hell, yes! The key to living with less pain is understanding what relieves pain, why it works, and how to achieve it.

Sometimes, the pain myths fed to us by society or family members suggest that we are the only ones with pain — that we are somehow broken and destined to live a painful life. Throughout the book, we will look at some of these ingrained stories, debunk them with data, and write constructive, true versions. Here is an example:

> **Myth:** I am the only one suffering with pain, and I will always have severe pain.
> **Fact:** One in five adult Americans report pain every day.
> **Relief-5R Approach:** Pain is common, and the Relief-5R plan can reduce and prevent it.

Current Pain Treatments and Their Deficiencies

The US healthcare system is designed to handle emergencies. It manages life-threatening heart attacks and acute fractures well. Thankfully, it saves lives. But most ongoing medical conditions are not life threatening, they are life draining. They chip away at joy. Ongoing painful conditions such as spine and arthritis pain steal people's daily lives. They limit the ability to stand up at a wedding, watch a child's soccer game from the sidelines, and even fetch the mail. Unfortunately, the medical system usually offers no lasting solutions.

Chronic painful conditions often have complex, interrelated

causes. Conventional healthcare is modeled around identifying and "fixing" an immediate and dangerous problem, not diagnosing and alleviating chronic painful conditions. If your pain continues beyond an "expected" course, or you want to avoid pain medications, or your pain occurs without a triggering event, then the current model fails. It fails to consider the whole person. It fails to address the imbalances fueling pain and dysfunction.

Insurance companies, hospital systems, and administrators push for algorithms to treat patients in a cookie-cutter way. This approach has some benefits. Standardized checklists and guidelines for treatment, for instance, help ensure that nothing is overlooked. Measuring outcomes helps assess the effectiveness of treatments. Standardization also identifies opportunities to save money and increase efficiency. But strict adherence to these algorithms, with little consideration of a person's unique medical history, lifestyle factors, and environment, results in subpar pain care. To minimize pain, eliminate suffering, and enable a person to function better, clinicians must see the whole person, reviewing their daily habits, activities, and environment alongside their medical history, physical exam, and diagnostic tests. These individual factors influence pain, disease, unease, and wellness.

In the current healthcare system, time and financial constraints have led to a divide-and-conquer attitude. Well-meaning physicians are allotted only ten to fifteen minutes for office visits, forcing them to focus on one issue and refer the patient to specialists to address additional concerns. A person with pain may be sent to a psychiatrist for depression, a lung doctor to assess sleep problems, and a cardiologist to treat high blood pressure. These specialists play an important role, but we need to remember that these conditions are interconnected. Seeing a person as a set of separate organ systems, and deciding on treatments (primarily medications) solely based on the assessment of a single system, fails to treat the source of the problem. We must consider the big picture: the whole, interconnected person.

Many prescription medication commercials tell us, "When diet and exercise fail, you can take this pill!" Ironically, this is an admission by the pharmaceutical industry that changes to our lifestyle (such as diet and exercise) are the first step to feeling better! It's also an admission that these changes can make medications unnecessary. Yet more than 68 percent of Americans receive at least one prescription medication every year. Ninety percent of Americans over age 65 take prescription medications, and almost 40 percent take more than five prescription medications.

While some medications are life-saving and necessary, the unintended effects of this smorgasbord of medications on multiple organ systems and the gut microbiome (discussed in chapter 3), in addition to known side effects, drug interactions, and cost, are mind-blowing. Many of these lab-synthesized chemicals may contribute to whole-body inflammation, stress, hormonal imbalances, gut damage, and impaired cognition, in addition to causing side effects that require many columns of small print to disclose. Yet medications are often considered the go-to treatment for both pain and inflammation. While pain and inflammation are undeniably linked — as inflammation levels rise, pain increases — medications are not the answer. They do not provide lasting relief.

Many of us can reduce the number and quantity of prescription medications we need by caring for our bodies. Research has shown that diet and other lifestyle changes could prevent 80 percent of inflammatory conditions such as diabetes, stroke, and premature heart disease. Inflammation drives these conditions and drives ongoing pain. To stop ongoing pain, we must reduce painful inflammation.

For decades, my colleagues and I have seen different people with the same MRI findings of severe back arthritis (severe stenosis). One person may have acute, piercing pain and have difficulty even walking to the bathroom. Another may have only mild pain and be surprised to learn that they have severe stenosis. Why does the same diagnosis produce such different symptoms? The differences arise from each person's unique combination of genetics, medical history, and fuel. *Fuel* refers not only to what we eat and drink but also to behavioral factors that feed into our well-being, such as exercise, sleep, stressors, and relationships. This combination determines an individual's overall level of painful inflammation. The good news is that some of these factors are within our control (figure 1.1).

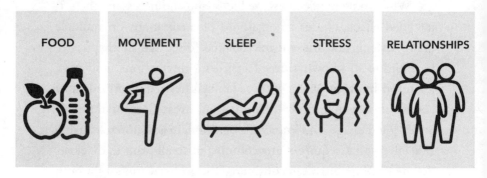

**Figure 1.1. Modifiable factors contributing to
chronic pain and inflammation.**

We become what we consume — and what we do. If we are stuck in a pattern of eating foods, practicing behaviors, and living in an environment that aggravates inflammation, then our body turns into a house of pain. If we break free of these patterns and improve our fuel, behaviors, and environment, we quell that inflammation. We can control our future with the choices we make today. For example, even if we have a strong family history of an inflammatory condition such as type 2 diabetes, we are not inevitably destined to have the disease. Our fuel, behaviors, and environment also play a role in determining whether we travel down a path of inflammation. These choices determine whether we become the best possible version of ourselves (figure 1.2). We must fuel well to feel well and be well.

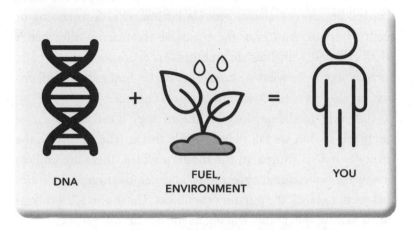

Figure 1.2. Key factors determining health and wellness.

The Holy Grail of medicine used to be increasing lifespan: now the goal is increasing healthspan, the number of years lived in good health with the ability to participate in life. Isn't this what we really want? Eighty years is a long lifespan, but if it is burdened by forty years of disease, a poor quality of life, and limited function, then the result is a short healthspan. Low back pain, neck pain, musculoskeletal disorders, and arthritis decrease healthspan.

Diet and lifestyle factors affect healthspan. A 2020 study published in the *Journal of the American Medical Association* found that maintaining a healthy weight, being physically active, not smoking, and limiting alcohol intake increased healthy years. Nutritious foods help extend our healthspan, as do improvements in physical activity, sleep, resilience, and healthy relationships.

In my medical training, we were taught five ways to treat pain: lifestyle modifications, physical therapy, medications, injections, and surgery. Lifestyle modifications are positive changes in diet, exercise, sleep, and stress levels. This is the first-line treatment for painful inflammation. Yet we tend to overlook this option in favor of tools that produce quicker results. Passive treatments (medications, injections, some surgeries) can relieve acute pain or nerve damage but do not always provide lasting relief for ongoing or recurring pain. And even these passive treatments work better when coupled with lifestyle changes. To decrease chronic pain, we must consider what we consume. Better fuel reduces inflammation, improves function, and restores balance.

Lifestyle medicine doctors like to say, "Diet and exercise rarely fail us, but we fail them." While this is true in theory, the reality is not so simple. In the modern world, there are endless pressures, professional obligations, and personal responsibilities that seem to block the pursuit of wellness. These obstacles sink us into a painful quicksand, leaving us unsure how to escape.

Freedom lies in taking little steps. By integrating small wellness changes into our chaotic days, we can stop suffering. The keys are discovering *what* would help, *why* these wellness choices matter, and *how* to incorporate them into a busy life. Understanding the *why* and the *how* are critical to living a life with less pain.

What would your life look like with more ease? Why do you want to prevent painful inflammation? What does *better* look like? If pain did not limit you, what activities would you do? What activities do you want to keep doing? Even if pain limits you from fully participating in one of your favorite activities, envision yourself doing it, and keep this mental image with you as your goal.

Pick meaningful goals for you (perhaps similar to the examples below, perhaps unique to you) and write them down. Make this book your own personal experiment.

- walking my dog
- picking up a child without severe pain
- going to a baseball game

- going shopping
- practicing yoga
- attending family events with more ease
- participating in my community
- doing volunteer work
- preventing severe pain

After picking your activity goals, break them down into things you need to work toward and things you can start doing now. For example, if hiking is one of your goals but walking is currently difficult for you, you might go to a place where you would like to hike, and walk around the trail entrance, complete a small portion of the trail, or simply envision yourself doing it. With that small step, a little taste of your future, you will be closer to your goal and eager to build on your progress.

You may also have broader, longer-term goals: being a healthy and active role model for your children, building your resilience, or working toward a personal or professional objective with less pain. The next chapter explains the basis of my Relief-5R plan. Chapters 3–7 each discuss one of the five individual pillars of the plan and set out a wide range of small lifestyle changes. After reading each chapter, choose the microboost changes that will fit in your life. Review your progress regularly to see how these small steps are bringing you closer to achieving your goals.

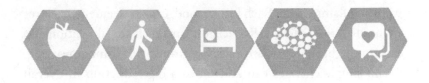

CHAPTER 2

The Relief-5R Plan

*In many cases, the outcome you want will continue
to elude you — even if you try harder.
But it may be possible if you try differently.
Can your current choices carry you to your desired future?
If not, something has to change. You can't get there from here.
You have to get on a different trajectory.*

— JAMES CLEAR

Modern life brims with little and big stressors, from never-ending phone notifications and late nights to the loss of a job or a devastating injury. These physical, mental, and emotional stressors intensify orthopaedic pain. They tighten our muscles, constrict blood vessels, and pinch nerves. When we are stressed, we become smaller, self-focused, and limited. Our bodies crumple into a ball of tension, inflammation, and pain, sometimes so bad that we have trouble standing up straight or walking.

The tools in this book can help you reduce painful inflammation and chronic stress in order to function and live better. What we fuel our bodies with today determines our future level of painful inflammation. Each bite of food, each movement, each response to stress, each sleep decision, and each social relationship can tip the balance toward or away from painful inflammation. Small, simple changes can add up to a big reduction in overall pain and inflammation, and a big increase in wellness. To understand how and why they work, let's look at some of the root causes of pain and the ways our body and brain send and interpret pain signals.

Lower Back Pain and Arthritis (Joint) Pain

More than 60 million Americans have had a recent bout of back pain. The leading causes of back pain include muscle sprains, spasms, degenerative disc disease, disc herniations, nerve root pinching, spinal stenosis (arthritis), facet joint spondylosis (arthritis), bony misalignments, abnormal spinal curvatures, and fractures. Disc herniations are a common cause of back pain. Spinal discs act as rubbery shock absorbers between the vertebrae (the bones of the spine). We can think of them as being like jelly donuts, with thicker outer layers and gelatinous middles. If there is a tear in the outer layer, some of the gelatinous substance may leak out: this is called a herniation. If this rupture occurs near a nerve, it may irritate the nerve and cause symptoms such as leg pain, weakness, and numbness. Arthritic bone spurs and cysts can also pinch nerves and cause similar symptoms (figure 2.1).

Other common sources of back pain are sacroiliac joint pain, bursitis, hip pain, piriformis syndrome, inflammatory arthritis, and widespread pain conditions like fibromyalgia. Some of these conditions can occur in combination. Other, less common forms of pain are related to conditions such as infection or cancer (and this is the reason that any ongoing pain must be evaluated by your physician).

With age, everybody develops some arthritic joint changes

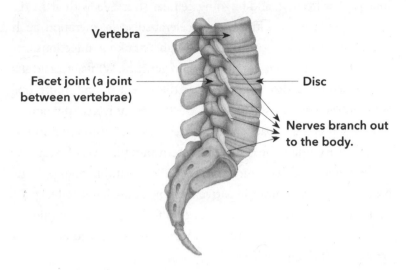

Figure 2.1. Lumbar (low back) anatomy.

as a result of wear and tear, but these can be aggravated by physical stressors, injuries, obesity, and genetics. Another risk factor is metabolic syndrome, which is a cluster of inflammatory abnormalities, including abdominal obesity, high blood sugar, high cholesterol, and high blood pressure. As these risk factors increase, so do inflammatory levels. Inflammation leads to cartilage breakdown and bony overgrowth in the joints and spine. But typical degenerative joint changes do not result in severe, debilitating pain for everybody, so what accounts for the difference? The answer is a combination of fuel and genetics. We cannot control aging or fully control our genetic risk factors, but we can control how we fuel our bodies.

Lumbar degenerative disc disease (wear and tear on the discs between our vertebrae) is one of the most commonly diagnosed causes of back pain and one for which treatment options are limited and often ineffective. Even the diagnosis of this pain is difficult, since it can be caused by multiple factors, including aging, injury, poor healing, and ongoing cellular stress. As with arthritis, certain risk factors are known to accelerate disc degeneration, such as physical trauma, carrying extra weight, smoking, infections, inflammation, metabolic conditions, and genetics. While most adults experience some disc degeneration, the extent of and, more important, the pain associated with this nearly universal phenomenon vary greatly. In particular, the degree of inflammation in the tissues surrounding the disc often determines the level of pain.

Furthermore, chronic painful inflammation changes our brains. It makes us more sensitive to pain: we are liable to feel pain even in response to light touch and to feel it beyond the injured area. Like a wildfire, painful inflammation can spread and grow stronger if it is left unchecked.

Fortunately, some of the risk factors for orthopaedic pain and inflammation are within our control, including daily food intake, activity level, sleep quality, mental stressors, and emotional stressors. To improve spine health and reduce pain, we must opt for real food, move more, use good ergonomics, sleep better, reduce stress, and focus on positive relationships. We can make these changes in bite-sized chunks and without time-consuming workouts, personal yoga instructors, or other costly or disruptive lifestyle changes.

Conventional pain treatment focuses on physical stress. Yet we know that mental and emotional stress worsen pain. Even without a definitive physical injury, mental and emotional stress can manifest as pain, spasms, and suffering. As an example, simply think about a corrupt politician, cutthroat coworker, or challenging family member. Picture the lines of their face, the sound of their voice, their negative words ringing in your ears, and the devastation caused by their actions. These thoughts may trigger tightness in your jaw, shoulders, or back. Your heart rate may quicken as your stress response flicks on.

Now take a big breath in and a longer breath out. Do this three more times. Then let out an audible, teenage-angst sigh. Now picture somebody you love — a family member, friend, mentor, or pet. Remember how you feel in their presence, the sound of their voice, and their warmth. You may notice some of the tightness melt away. This experience reminds us that the mind and body are not separate entities: what happens in the mind manifests in the body and vice versa. Simply put, all forms of stress contribute to inflammation and pain (figure 2.2).

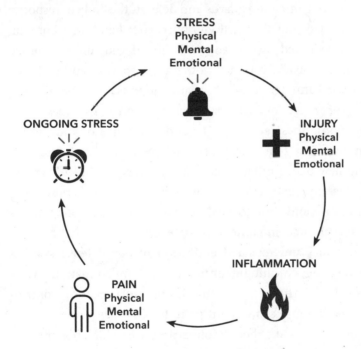

Figure 2.2. Stress cycle and pain with or without an injury.

Inflammation and Pain

Our body strives to maintain balance, or *homeostasis*, to survive without overresponding to all the stimuli in our constantly changing environment. To keep this balance, our body has multiple feedback loops. A threat, such as an injury, infection, or dangerous situation, activates our defense systems to release stress hormones, increase our heart rate, raise our blood pressure, and prepare us to run or fight. These systems are designed to stay activated for short periods until we have escaped or neutralized the threat; then the body returns to its equilibrium. Continuous exposure to physical, mental, and emotional stressors results in ongoing activation of our defense systems. This in turn leads to increased inflammation and more pain signaling.

Acute inflammation guards and defends the body in response to an injury or imbalance. If you burn your hand on a hot pan, the area turns red, swells, and feels hot. If you suffer a muscle strain in your back, you may notice pain, spasms, and swelling. The classic Latin definition of inflammation is *dolor* (pain), *calor* (heat), *rubor* (redness), *tumor* (swelling), and *functio laesa* (loss of function). These are the signs and symptoms of your body's inflammatory system at work, removing damaged cells and generating new ones. Initially, these are good signs. But if signs of inflammation persist after the injury has been given appropriate medical care and time to heal, it may be because your body is stuck in a chronic, inflammatory state.

Poor fuel and repeated activation of our defense systems cause ongoing, chronic inflammation. The inflammation switch gets stuck "on" (figure 2.3). This chronic inflammation contributes to back, muscle, and joint pain. It also plays a role in autoimmune diseases like rheumatoid arthritis, in which the immune system attacks the body itself, and common, serious conditions such as heart disease and diabetes.

Inflammation, Pain, and Excess Fat

Excess body fat disrupts the body's homeostasis. It adds to physical stress, disturbs spine and joint alignment, and results in the

NORMAL INFLAMMATION   **CHRONIC INFLAMMATION**

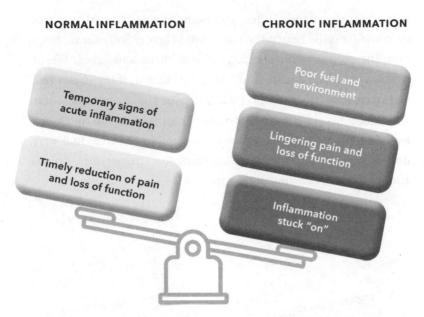

Figure 2.3. Normal vs. chronic inflammation.

production of more inflammatory substances in the body, including interleukin-6 (IL-6), tumor necrosis factor alpha (TNF-α), and C-reactive protein (CRP). An especially dangerous type of fat is extra belly fat. Belly fat is not an inert blob; it consists of active cells that produce inflammatory molecules such as TNF-α and IL-6. They pump out signals that tip the whole body toward a state of painful inflammation. This can lead to early back arthritis, more joint pain, more muscle pain, autoimmune diseases, diabetes, heart disease, and other conditions — all of which further stress the body. The kicker is that chronic stress causes our bodies to cling to extra fat, creating an unending cycle of inflammation. We must address physical, mental, and emotional stressors together to alleviate inflammation.

The pain-signaling pathways in our body are another form of defense. The acute pain of touching a hot pan triggers you to withdraw your hand. When you remove the external cause of pain and treat the injury, the pain should abate. Sometimes, however, the pain lingers — it pierces and burns and aches. Weeks later, pain signals continue to flood the brain as if the injury had just occurred. If left unchecked, the pain signals are amplified, and your body misinterprets sensory information: the touch of a feather may feel painful, and a prickly pain engulfs areas that were not injured. The pain switch gets stuck "on" (figure 2.4). This is another result of chronic inflammation.

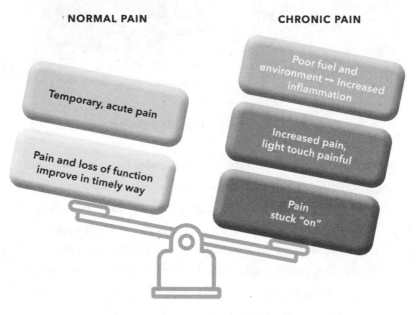

Figure 2.4. Normal vs. chronic pain.

The Stress System (Sympathetic Nervous System)

If your body perceives a threat to survival (a lion, fire, or robber), it signals your body's acute stress response, known as the sympathetic (fight-or-flight) response. This causes a release of adrenaline, cortisol, and other hormones to prepare your body to protect itself. These hormones cause your heart rate and blood pressure to spike. Your muscles tense, ready to fight or flee — or, sometimes, freeze. You become hyperalert but unable to focus. Your eyes dilate, blood is shunted to your large muscles, your blood sugar rises, goose bumps erupt, and your immune system goes haywire. Nonemergency systems like higher thinking, digestion, and bladder control slow down as your body's resources are diverted to survival systems. You are pumped up to fight or run for your life.

Once the acute threat is gone, the stress response normally stops. It is designed to be activated for brief emergencies. But now imagine that this stress response is activated multiple times a day by mundane stressors like sitting in traffic, dealing with difficult people at work, meeting unrealistic deadlines, arguing with family members, and constantly multitasking. In a dangerous situation, the stress response protects us, but repeated activation hurts us. The fight-or-flight response gets stuck "on" (figure 2.5). In this state of chronic stress, we are hyperalert and irritable but unable to concentrate. Our muscles tense, our blood sugar rises, and our immune system (our defense) turns on us. This system overdrive prevents clear thinking and optimal functioning. Even worse, it damages our bodies and results in more painful inflammation. It must be reset and rebalanced.

A stressful event or injury can tense muscles all over your body. Think of a whiplash car injury. Your neck jerks back and forth, unprepared for the impact, and then locks into spasm. The surrounding muscles turn rock-hard. Your entire spine stiffens. After a few weeks pass, assuming that a medical examination has ruled out serious injury, your neck muscles should start to loosen with the assistance of stretches, heat, and possibly physical therapy or a short course of medication. But if you are experiencing ongoing stress and poor fuel, you may experience continued

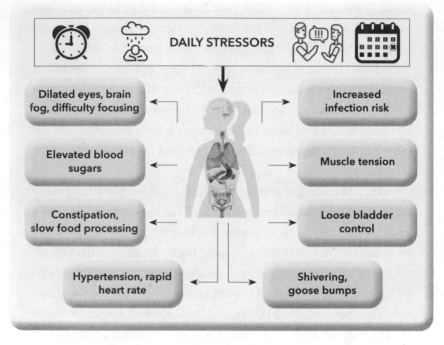

Figure 2.5. Chronic stress response.

tension, pain, and suffering. Chronic activation shifts our entire body into a state of stress, pain, and inflammation. The defense systems all get stuck "on" (figure 2.6).

The Problems with Medications

If pain and inflammation overdrive worsen back, muscle, and joint pain, why not simply take medications to block these systems? Healthcare providers routinely recommend nonsteroidal anti-inflammatory drugs (NSAIDs), opioids (narcotics), and steroids for pain. If your body is injured or inflamed, the pain is a message from your brain: "Something is wrong, please fix this!" The message is not "Please muzzle the messenger for a few hours." Yet that is the effect of these medications. The pharmaceutical

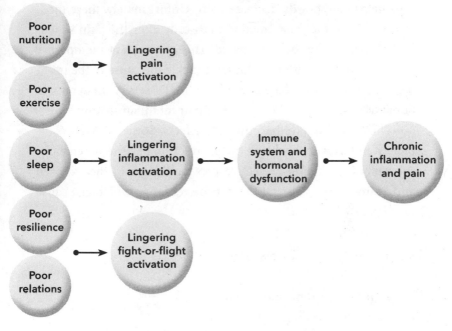

Figure 2.6. Lifestyle factors causing chronic, painful inflammation.

industry promotes the fantasy of zero pain: take a pill and eliminate pain. But pills offer only temporary, superficial relief and often have adverse effects. Let's look at how these common pain medications work and why they are not the best way to manage chronic pain.

NSAIDs

NSAIDs are commonly and liberally prescribed for the relief of orthopaedic pain and other inflammatory conditions with pain, stiffness, and swelling. When a tissue injury or infection occurs, cells release inflammatory substances called cytokines. NSAIDs such as ibuprofen (Advil), naproxen (Aleve), and aspirin block the production of cytokines, including interleukins and TNF-α.

This helps temporarily decrease pain. Unfortunately, these medications block the inflammation path only after the pain signaling mechanism has been activated. This approach is a temporary Band-aid, not a solution. It does not tackle the cause of the problem. Treatment of chronic pain with NSAIDs sets us up to remain dependent and trapped in a cycle of painful inflammation.

NSAIDs also have harmful side effects. Some NSAIDs completely and irreversibly block the production of certain beneficial substances, including protective prostaglandins in the stomach and kidneys. They disrupt the gut microbiome, which can cause more pain.

SOME SIDE EFFECTS OF NSAIDs
- acid reflux
- stomach bleeding and ulcers
- intestinal bleeding
- kidney disease
- nausea, vomiting, and diarrhea
- rash and other allergic reactions
- slower healing of injuries to tendons, ligaments, and bones
- kidney damage
- liver damage
- increased risk of heart attack and stroke

Opioids

Opioids, such as hydrocodone, oxycodone, and morphine, are commonly prescribed to relieve pain after an acute injury or major surgery. But the pharmaceutical promotion of "zero pain" and other factors have led patients to expect prescriptions for opioids after smaller surgeries, such as a hernia repair, gallbladder removal, or appendix removal. A 2020 study reveals that 91 percent of patients in the United States are prescribed opioids after these surgeries, compared with only 5 percent of patients in other countries.

While opioids may be of value in the initial days after a fracture or major surgery, beyond this period the harms outweigh the benefits. Opioid use can lead to rebound pain (when the opioid wears off) and increased pain signals over time. The suppressed pain message changes from a wimpy, indoor voice to a loud, outdoor voice. There is even a phenomenon called *opioid-induced hyperalgesia*, which makes people taking opioids more sensitive than other people to painful stimuli. In other words, a little needle poke to the shoulder feels like the blow of a fiery sword to the entire arm.

Opioids activate reward centers in the brain and cause a release of endorphins. These are neurotransmitters that make the mind and body feel good. They reduce pain and boost pleasure. The problem is that once the medication stops working, the mind and body may start to crave the good feelings and easy pick-me-ups. This leads to the danger of addiction. Even if we do not develop cravings, over time the body develops a tolerance to opioids and requires more medication to produce the same effect. Recent research has shown that this is in part because long-term use of opioids increases painful inflammation. Opioids negatively affect multiple body systems. Their depressive effects slow breathing and impair digestion, heart function, and cognitive functions, causing brain fog and leading to falls and other accidents. Multiple studies have confirmed a higher rate of fractures for people taking opioids.

Opioids disrupt hormone balances, affecting sexual and reproductive function as well as mood. Some research shows that these hormonal changes can also lead to prediabetes and more inflammation. In light of the recent pandemic, another key concern is that opioids suppress the immune system. Multiple studies have found that people who take opioids over a long period have worse overall health outcomes. Clearly, opioids wreak havoc on the human body even without taking into account the risks of addiction, overdose, and death, and the associated social harms.

SOME SIDE EFFECTS OF OPIOIDS

- depressed breathing
- sleep apnea
- constipation and risk of bowel obstruction
- decreased sexual function and fertility
- increased risk of falls and fractures
- foggy thinking
- increased pain and pain sensitivity
- addiction
- depression
- impaired immune system
- increased risk of heart failure

Steroids

Steroids, such as prednisone, block the same inflammation pathway as NSAIDs, but at an earlier point. They are powerful drugs used to reduce inflammation in the case of an acute injury or to blunt a dangerous immune response, such as an intense allergic reaction. But long-term use results in potentially severe effects on multiple body systems. Steroids are not a long-term pain solution.

SOME SIDE EFFECTS OF LONG-TERM STEROID USE

- osteoporosis
- muscle and joint damage
- stomach ulcers
- leg cramps

- increased body hair growth
- hypertension, rapid heart rate
- mood swings, anger, depression
- insomnia
- fluid retention, electrolyte imbalances, and kidney problems
- diabetes
- adrenal damage
- increased risk of infections

Our goal is to restore balance, not cause more chaos. Medications may temporarily decrease back, joint, and muscle pain, but they do not treat the root cause. Even worse, most pills create more imbalances and result in bigger problems. There is a better way.

The Relief-5R Alternative to Pain Medications

If all these widely prescribed medications come at such a cost to our physical and mental health, what alternatives do we have for relief from chronic pain? The Relief-5R plan saves our bodies from chronic painful inflammation, improves overall health, and restores quality of life. This is my prescription for you to ease back, muscle, and joint pain (figure 2.7).

Setting Goals

The Relief 5R-plan is simple and free, but it does require commitment to the goal of living with less pain. The secret to achieving goals is breaking them down into small steps and taking the first little step. We stand the best chance of succeeding when we write down our goals, make them specific, break them into small, actionable steps, and hold ourselves accountable. A goal like "I will

DR. SHARMA'S Rx PAD

Crush pain and inflammation with the Relief-5R plan

- **Refuel** with natural, unprocessed food
- **Revitalize** through regular movement
- **Recharge** through restorative sleep
- **Refresh** by building resilience
- **Relate** by connecting with others

Cost: Free

Quantity and refill: Unlimited

No side effects

Evidence-based

Figure 2.7. Dr. Sharma's prescription for
back, muscle, and joint pain.

eat more plant-based foods" is a setup for failure — it is broad, nonspecific, and offers no path for getting from where you are to where you want to be.

The pathway to success consists of specific, small changes in your routine to help you feel better and form lasting, beneficial habits. These *microboosts* are little steps that boost you toward ease and relief. In the past you may have found it difficult to make changes because they were not tailored to the way you live. Unfortunately, willpower alone is not enough to build lasting change. We must create habits that fit our individual lives.

An effective way to work toward your goals is to use a method called *implementation intention.* It means creating a plan that specifies the *who, what, why, when, where,* and *how* of working toward your goal. We know you (the *who*) want to crush painful inflammation (the *what*) to live better (the *why*). The microboosts recommended in this book show you the *how.* Deciding *when* and *where* you will implement your chosen microboosts builds a realistic, customized pain relief plan.

Microboosts work best when they are part of our established daily activities, such as eating dinner, brushing our teeth, and driving to work. Adding a visual cue helps reinforce the new behavior. To make it stick, articulate your active, concrete microboosts aloud and in writing. Each morning and evening, review your microboosts and big goals.

The human brain loves rewards, and seeing evidence of progress motivates us not only to stick with it but to do more. Log your progress daily and review it weekly. For every day you filled half your dinner plate with vegetables, substituted berries for a processed dessert, or passed up a bag of chips for a handful of nuts, add a penny to a jar, a sticker to a calendar, or a check to a phone application. If you complete your microboosts for a week, reward yourself with a special outing or healthy treat!

Success also requires removing roadblocks, pitfalls, deterrents, and distractions. For example, if you are trying to increase your activity level after work, but you know that once you start watching television you will not exercise later, then move the remote control to another room, or lay your workout clothes on the couch the night before. Place a sticky note on the clothes with your written goal and a reminder to hit the play button on your workout playlist *now.* Make it easy to follow the pain-relief path.

It's also important to recognize what triggers unhealthy choices. If you know, for instance, that eating one cookie will inevitably mean that you eat three more, you have various options.

You could remove all cookies from the house. You could allow yourself one cookie a day and put it in a container labeled by the day of the week. Or you could keep real food front and center, with the cookies out of sight. Think of it like setting up a store — keep all the things you want to focus on at eye level and attractively displayed. It is also powerful and motivating to say and write "I" statements, such as "I will have berries for dessert after dinner." This reinforces your intention and helps it sink in as *your* plan, not just an idea. Use the mnemonic *RELIEF* to find easy ways to add microboosts to your day.

R	<u>R</u>emove barriers
E	<u>E</u>ye level
L	<u>L</u>ink to a specific activity
I	"<u>I</u>" declaration
E	<u>E</u>ncourage progress by tracking
F	<u>F</u>eel better!

Next Steps

1. Decide to build a lifestyle for less pain, less stress, and increased function.
2. Use the Relief-5R plan to reach your personal goals and live the life you deserve.
3. Make customized changes in your daily routine that add up to big pain relief.
4. Feel better!

CHAPTER 3

Refuel

If it came from a plant, eat it; if it was made in a plant, don't.
— MICHAEL POLLAN

Myth: Orthopaedic pain is not affected by food choices.
Fact: Food programs the body for more or less pain and inflammation.
Relief-5R: Optimizing our fuel is part of a pain solution.

Food and orthopaedic pain may not seem linked. In fact, most orthopaedists recommend medications, injections, and surgery for pain relief, not a pain-fighting food plan. This approach ignores a major pain factor. The standard American diet (SAD) is full of foods that aggravate pain: added sugar, excess salt, unhealthy fats, and artificial ingredients. The SAD triggers painful inflammation. Processed foods, the crown jewels of the SAD, are found everywhere, from our workplaces and schools to convenience stores, fast-food restaurants, and hospitals. Even when we know they are not healthy, they trap us into wanting more. This is no accident. The food industry designs these highly processed foods to trigger the reward system in our brains, just like opioids! They want to trigger what they call a "bliss point," an exact ratio of extra sugar, salt, and fat that gives us a high and creates cravings. This is *sick*.

The industry exploits more than just our sense of taste. An award-winning scientific study, dubbed the "sonic chip" study, revealed that the louder the crunch of a chip when we bite into it, the more fresh, crispy, and desirable we perceive it to be. This trickery hijacks the feel-good signals in the brain to make eating a processed chip feel like eating a crisp, ripe apple. Through no fault of our own, we are duped into craving these substances. Processed food is quick, cheap, and emotionally rewarding. Trillions of dollars a year are spent on advertising to keep us coming back for more. It seems nearly impossible to escape the processed-food trap on our own. It's not because we lack willpower. It is because we are under *a biological attack*.

But armed with a plan for healthy refueling, we can break free. First, we must recognize that how we fuel our bodies determines how well we function. Our fuel and environment can build us up or break us down. They determine our inflammation and pain levels. Smart nutrition choices can help heal damage to our bodies and prevent future degeneration. Nourishing food activates natural pain-control mechanisms in the body and helps us more efficiently clean out wastes and harmful substances. It can reduce painful inflammation in our spine, joints, and muscles. Studies have shown that consuming real, unprocessed food reduces pain, inflammation, and cellular damage. Each food decision tips the balance toward or away from painful inflammation. Once freed from the hooks of processed food, we get to choose. We can quell and prevent pain with better food choices. Let's dig in! We will start with an overview of the typical diet and its connection to chronic pain, look at easy ways to improve our food intake, and discover practical ways to add microboosts to our day.

My Refuel Experience

Everything I thought was rewarding me was poisoning me. A busy shift, a difficult morning, or a sluggish feeling called for a diet soda. The bubbles danced on my tongue and reenergized me — without sugar. A win, I thought. Little did I know that diet soda intake correlates with higher rates of inflammation, diabetes, and metabolic syndrome, that diet soda consumption is associated with a greater risk of kidney failure, or that both sugar-sweetened and diet soft drinks are linked with obesity. It gets worse. During the afternoon slump, I would gobble down processed cookies or candy and be puzzled in the evening when a food baby erupted. My treats — soda, processed food, and simple carbohydrates — were fueling destructive inflammation. I was unknowingly hurting myself.

It was not until I was pregnant that I began making connections between my diet and my health. When I developed gestational diabetes (diabetes of pregnancy), I was shocked, since I was at a healthy weight and exercised regularly. Through this diagnosis I came face to face with my family history of diabetes. I resolved to make lifestyle changes to manage my blood sugar, reduce inflammation, and ensure the safety of my growing bundle of joy.

For the first time in my life, I learned how to use nutritional labels. I found that my blood sugar was better controlled if I ate more fiber, adequate protein, and no fake, fat-free foods. Four times a day, I stabbed my fingertip to measure my blood sugar and discovered how it was affected by my food choices and activity level. An afternoon walk lowered my blood sugar enough that I could enjoy a fun-size candy bar afterward. At a New Year's Day brunch, I learned I could eat a donut with two strips of bacon on top and not bump my blood sugar (though I don't recommend it — more on this later). How could I be a physician and know so little about this? I knew I couldn't be the only one.

The Standard American Diet

Only 1.5 percent of Americans consume an ideal diet, as reported by the American Heart Association. The standard American diet (SAD) is more than sad; it breeds pain, inflammation, and disease. It is composed of processed foods high in added sugar, added salt, and saturated fats, and low in nutrients. It lacks vegetables, fruits, and legumes. This processed, nutrient-poor diet increases pain and inflammation.

SAD Effects

- increased inflammation
- increased pain
- increased recovery time from painful injuries
- increased pain flares
- increased fat mass
- decreased lean body mass

Poor nutrition drives poor health. It contributes to heart disease, diabetes, obesity, and certain cancers. It fans the flames of inflammation, causing pain in our spine, joints, and muscles. Thankfully, we can calm the inferno with better nutrition choices.

Over the years, our society's food intake has shifted from locally grown and home-cooked meals to processed, nutrient-poor, calorie-rich, and preservative-filled meals and drinks. How did we get here? The shift began decades ago as the food industry perfected the taste of addictive artificial flavors, World War II changed food availability and family dynamics, frozen TV dinners were created, salt consumption rose, lobbyists pushed their food products, and agricultural subsidies for corn motivated the addition of inexpensive corn syrup to all sorts of processed foods.

Real Food: Unprocessed and Naked

Real food is a term that is thrown around a lot. Ideally, it means one-ingredient, unprocessed food. These real foods are the foods we should buy, eat, and cook with. Processed foods are pumped full of chemicals to make them taste, look, smell, sound, and feel like real food. The additives in a bag of chips or a box of factory-made baked "goods"— artificial colors, sugar, salt, artificial sweeteners, and fillers — activate the body's stress response and aggravate pain, inflammation, and disease. When your body is trying to fight the fire of inflammation, let's not douse it with kerosene.

Real food shifts your body to relief mode. It does not need additives to make it look, smell, taste, feel, and sound like the real thing. It *is* the real thing. It provides protective antioxidants, nourishes your good gut bacteria, decreases your risk of disease, and lowers painful inflammation.

While some may say real food costs more than chemical-laden food, and many people may not have easy access to fresh food, there are still simple ways to eat real food, such as purchasing frozen real foods, "ugly" produce (slightly misshapen produce often offered at cheaper prices), and seasonally abundant foods. Additionally, legumes such as chickpeas, kidney beans, and black beans are less expensive than most processed foods. In the long-term, eating real food saves your body from painful inflammation and saves money by reducing healthcare bills.

The Food Pyramid

The changes in national dietary recommendations over time visually encapsulate the sad shift to the SAD. Dietary recommendations from the United States Department of Agriculture (USDA) in the 1940s provided better guidance than the infamous 1992 food pyramid (figure 3.1). The 1940s food wheel recommended eating from each of seven food groups daily to ensure a nutritious diet. It emphasized plant food loaded with phytonutrients rich in antioxidant and anti-inflammatory effects. The first three numeric groups consist of nutrient-dense foods, including leafy green vegetables, citrus fruits, tomatoes, and raw cabbage. The wheel orders vegetables before fruits and notes the importance of raw, whole vegetables. The fourth group is dairy products, followed by meats, fish, and legumes. The last two groups are bread, flour, cereals, and margarine. Vegetables and fruits, including legumes (beans and peas), account for approximately half the wheel.

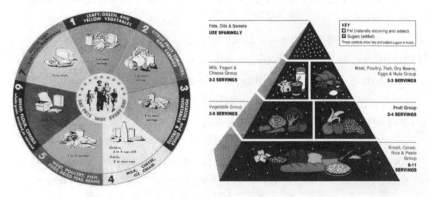

Figure 3.1. USDA 1940s wheel (left) and 1992 food pyramid.

In contrast, the 1992 food pyramid recommends a diet heavily based on carbohydrates such as breads, rice, and pasta, including highly processed foods. America listened. The increase in consumption of these foods paralleled rises in inflammatory pain, heart disease, diabetes, and the multilayered opioid crisis. While several factors contributed to the rise of processed foods, the 1992 food pyramid was instrumental in persuading people that inflammatory foods constituted a healthy diet.

Thankfully, food pyramids were put to rest in 2011 and replaced by a plate image. It recommends a plate half filled with whole fruits and vegetables, and half with whole grains and animal and plant protein sources (figure 3.2).

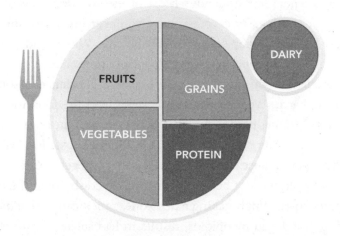

Figure 3.2. USDA 2011 MyPlate, www.myplate.gov.

This is a step in the right direction. Studies have found that switching from the SAD to a diet high in natural, unprocessed foods results in faster healing after an injury and prevents painful inflammation. In addition, a 2021 review of more than fifteen studies confirmed that a proinflammatory diet (like the SAD) increases feelings of distress, anxiety, and depression, which all worsen pain. In other words, better food fuels a healthier body with less pain and less inflammation. Let's get into why and how!

Sugar

As with opioids, Americans consume more sugar per person than people in any other country. Added sugar may be the most damning part of the SAD. High sugar intake is linked to nutritional imbalances, obesity, and several major diseases. By disrupting proper digestion, altering the gut microbiome, and contributing to inflammation, it causes major *dis-ease*. Yet even when we understand the harms of sugar, we crave it and have trouble limiting our intake. Ever binged on an entire bag of cookies? Mindlessly eaten a whole box of candy? Most of us have done this at one point or another. By contrast, have you ever uncontrollably devoured a bag of baby carrots? Probably not. When foods do not have addictive properties, we can control our intake.

Addiction means continued use of a substance despite it causing harm. We are addicted to sugar, and the food industry knows it. Studies have shown that sugar activates the reward pathway in our brain similarly to other addictive substances. We eat more sugar because it makes us feel good — we get a rush, a high, and an energy boost before the inevitable crash. Then the cycle repeats. Interestingly, taking naltrexone, a medication that blocks the high induced by opioids, results in less sugar consumption. Without the high, sugar loses its appeal.

Over time, as with other addictive substances, we develop a tolerance and need more sugar to satisfy our sweet tooth. Sugar actually changes our sense of taste. Freaky, right? A randomized controlled study divided people with the same baseline sugar intake into a low-sugar group and a second group with no change in sugar intake. After two months on these diets, both groups were offered the same dessert. The low-sugar group found the dessert sweeter than the group who had not changed their sugar intake. After three months, the low-sugar group rated the same dessert 40 percent sweeter than the other group.

Our sugar intake molds our own tastes and perceived needs. On the one hand, this means that without restricting the sugar we consume, we are likely to crave more and more of it. On the other, it means that we have the power to control that craving. We can free ourselves from sugar addiction and experience less inflammation and less pain.

I have experienced this shift firsthand. As a screening test for gestational diabetes, pregnant women undergo a glucose tolerance test, which requires drinking a highly concentrated glucose solution — a neon orange, slimy goo. During my first pregnancy, when I was consuming large quantities of sugar, I slurped it down like a 5-year-old eating birthday cake. Two years later, in my second pregnancy, I had difficulty even finishing the wretched goop. Reducing my sugar intake during and after my first pregnancy had normalized my taste preferences.

We learn early in life that sugar rots our teeth. What we often don't learn is that it rots our bodies and our brains as well. It pulls us into a downward spiral of inflammation, pain, depression, and brain fog. Little daily changes enable us to break out of this spiral. Since I put the kibosh on added sugar, I no longer get "hangry" (feeling so hungry that I become irritable), suffer from an afternoon slump, or wake up with upper back spasms. My taste buds appreciate natural food, and intermittent fasting feels easy. This is freedom — freedom from cravings, body aches, hunger pangs, and energy slumps. This is a better life with less painful inflammation.

SOME SIDE EFFECTS OF ADDED SUGAR
- energy slumps and irritability
- cravings
- brain fog
- mood swings and depression
- weight gain

- increased risk of diabetes
- more inflammation and inflammatory conditions

How much sugar should we consume, and how do we go about reducing our consumption? The first step is to reduce our intake of foods and drinks with added sugar. We can be mindful of foods that contain naturally high levels of sugar, such as whole fruits, but these are not the main culprits of inflammation. It is the added sugar that we have to limit.

A teaspoon of sugar is equivalent to about 4 grams. The American Heart Association recommends limiting added sugars to six teaspoons (about 25 grams) for women and nine teaspoons (37 grams) for men per day. This includes added sugars from all sources, including drinks (such as sweetened coffee, chai, sodas, and fruit juices). But the average American consumes more than twenty-two teaspoons (88 grams) of added sugar every day. A single can of cola contains 41 grams — well over the recommended daily limit for any adult.

One easy way to start, then, is to gradually stop adding sugar to tea or coffee and to avoid sweetened beverages. We can also reduce our consumption of foods we know to be high in sugar, such as those listed below.

Foods and Drinks High in Added Sugar

- baked goods (breads, cake, cookies)
- donuts
- chocolate, candy, marshmallows
- puddings, ice cream, sorbet
- sweetened coffee and tea, hot chocolate, mocha drinks, chocolate milk
- sports drinks, fruit juices, sodas
- jams, jellies, syrups

Part of the difficulty in moderating our sugar consumption, however, is that added sugar hides in a wide range of processed foods, including savory foods. While we may aspire to eat natural, unprocessed food most of the time, always preparing meals from scratch may not be realistic. But one serving of store-bought pasta sauce can have more than five grams of added sugar. At the grocery store, it's important to check product labels. Ideally, food products should consist of five or fewer ingredients that are all real foods and not sugar, chemicals, or additives.

Common Sources of Hidden Added Sugar

- packaged soups
- packaged cereals
- ready-made waffles, waffle and pancake mixes
- breads and crackers
- baby food
- yogurt
- salad dressing, ketchup, sauces, and other condiments
- cured meats
- pasta sauces
- creamy foods
- peanut butter

Okay, you'll check labels for added sugar — done deal, right? Not quite. The industry has one more trick up its sleeve: deceptive ingredient lists. As you may know, US food product labels list ingredients in descending order of quantity. The industry knows that listing sugar as the first ingredient will discourage consumers. They get around this by listing sugar in several different forms. For example, a bottle of barbecue sauce may list tomatoes as the first ingredient — sounds healthy, doesn't it? But the label may also list high-fructose corn syrup, honey, molasses, corn syrup, and sugar. Overall, sugar, in these various forms, is the most abundant ingredient. Sneaky. Deceptive. Sick and making us sicker. Avoid this painful sugar trap by looking out for the different forms of sugar listed below. Note that the suffix -*ose* in an ingredient list indicates a form of sugar. A balance of naturally occurring sugars in fruits and vegetables is fine; it is added sugar that we want to avoid.

SUGAR BY ANOTHER NAME

- agave
- brown sugar
- corn syrup or corn sweetener
- coconut sugar
- date sugar
- dextrose
- fructose
- fruit juice concentrate
- glucose
- high-fructose corn syrup
- honey
- invert sugar
- lactose
- malt
- maltose
- molasses
- sorbitol
- sucrose

Artificial sweeteners are not the answer either. Many artificial sweeteners have been shown to alter the gut microbiome and disrupt the immune system, leading to inflammation, obesity, and disease. *Just say no* to added sugar and sugar substitutes.

Fiber

We have dumped added sugar; now let's add pain-fighting foods high in healthy fiber. Before I lose you, I am not talking about 1980s fiber drinks! Dietary fiber is found in vegetables, fruits, beans, peas, legumes, nuts, seeds, and whole-grain foods — in other words, natural, unprocessed foods. Because it slows down the absorption of sugars and sates our appetite, it's a double win for lowering painful inflammation. Studies of thousands of people have found that greater fiber consumption results in less arthritic knee pain. Eat more fiber, have less joint pain? Sign me up! As a bonus, fiber reduces the risk of prolonged pain, metabolic syndrome, diabetes, and heart disease. Most unprocessed foods are good sources of fiber.

BENEFITS OF FIBER

- decreases pain and inflammation
- balances out sugar intake and prevents blood-sugar spikes
- quells hunger
- decreases risk of heart disease
- lowers blood pressure and cholesterol
- feeds the microbiome (good gut bacteria)
- maintains normal bowel movements

GOOD SOURCES OF FIBER

- **Whole grains:** Brown rice, quinoa, oats, corn, wild rice, whole-wheat bread and pasta, barley, wheat bran, oat bran
- **Legumes:** Lentils, soybeans, tofu, navy beans, chickpeas, kidney beans, black beans, lima beans, split peas, peas
- **Vegetables:** Carrots, artichokes, chard, beets, sweet potatoes, asparagus, turnips, brussels sprouts, okra, broccoli, cauliflower, cabbage, kale, spinach, bok choy, collard greens, radishes, rutabagas, watercress

- **Fruit:** Raspberries, avocados, apples, oranges, bananas, strawberries, blueberries, pears
- **Nuts and seeds:** Walnuts, almonds, hazelnuts, pecans, macadamia nuts, pistachios, pumpkin seeds, chia seeds, sunflower seeds, flaxseeds

Glycemic Index

The glycemic index (GI) is a measure of how quickly a food increases our blood sugar level after eating it. On a scale from 1 to 100, pure sugar ranks 100. High-GI foods (70–100) spike our blood sugar and contribute to pain, inflammation, and disease. Medium GI foods (56–59) cause a moderate rise in our blood sugars. Low-GI foods (1–55) cause a slower, steadier rise in blood sugar and can help reduce pain and inflammation. Typically, processed foods have a higher GI than unprocessed food and high-fiber foods, so it's not surprising that the list below overlaps with the list of high-fiber foods. GI serves as a guideline, but a low GI does not necessarily mean that a particular food is healthy; we still have to consider the other ingredients and be wary of added sugar and processed ingredients. Real food reigns supreme.

Lower-GI Foods
- **Vegetables:** Asparagus, avocados, broccoli, carrots, cauliflower, celery, cucumber, eggplant, green beans, lettuce, mushrooms, peas, spinach, squash, tomatoes, yams, zucchini
- **Fruits (whole, fresh):** Apples, apricots, berries, cherries, grapefruit, grapes, oranges, mangoes, peaches, pears, plums, strawberries
- **Legumes:** Baked beans, black beans, butter beans, cannellini beans, chickpeas, kidney beans, lentils, lima beans, peanuts, split peas

- **Pasta, noodles, rice, grains:** Barley, basmati rice, brown rice, buckwheat, cracked wheat, quinoa, pearl couscous, rice noodles, rolled oats, semolina pasta, soba noodles, vermicelli
- **Dairy products and nondairy alternatives:** Almond milk, cheese, custard, milk, soy milk, yogurt (with no or low added sugar)

VERY LOW-GI FOODS

- eggs
- fats and oils
- fish
- herbs

- meats
- nuts
- seafood
- spices

The idea is to eat primarily real, unprocessed food. Remember the 1940s food wheel? It was genius. If you want less pain, less inflammation, and less disease, focus on eating real food.

Phytonutrients

What if there were a super medicine that could boost health, charge the immune system, protect your joints, and fight inflammation with no side effects and little cost? Would you be interested? Yes? Well, it exists in the form of phytonutrients. Found in plants, phytonutrients are the chemicals that give plants their color, their protection against pests and diseases, and their strength. They are the plant's superpowers. For humans, phytonutrients act as antioxidants: they reduce and help to heal oxidative damage to our tissues and reduce inflammation. For example, the polyphenols found in berries, turmeric, and green tea help preserve our joints and limit arthritis damage. Studies have shown that an increased intake of polyphenol phytonutrients slows down joint and back degeneration, increases collagen production (important to skin and joint health), and decreases cell death (see figure 3.3). Carotenoids are another type of polyphenol. They are found in leafy greens, such as spinach, and orange plant foods, such as squash and sweet potatoes. Curcumin, found in turmeric, acts as an antioxidant and a natural NSAID. Polyphenols enhance our immune system, protect our eyesight, improve our skin, restore homeostasis, and shift our body to a healthier, low-inflammation state. What more could we ask for? These are pain-fighting super foods!

DIETARY POLYPHENOLS

↑ Joint strength
↓ Oxidative damage
↓ Cell death
↓ Arthritis degeneration
↓ Pain
↓ Inflammation

Figure 3.3. Effect of polyphenols on arthritis, pain, and inflammation.

Our bodies cannot produce these vital nutrients. We need to eat a variety of colorful plant foods to obtain them and *squash* painful inflammation (pun intended). Many are easily identified by the color of the food.

IMPORTANT PHYTONUTRIENTS
- **Carotenoids** (found in red, orange, yellow, and green plant foods)
  - Beta-carotene: found in dark, leafy greens and orange vegetables and fruits, such as broccoli, spinach, collard greens, kale, sweet potatoes, pumpkin, squash, and cantaloupe

- Lutein: found in greens such as lettuce, broccoli, kale, collard greens, brussels sprouts, and artichokes
- Lycopene: found in red and pink vegetables and fruits, such as red peppers, watermelon, tomatoes, and grapefruit
- **Polyphenols**
  - Resveratrol: found in blue and purple foods, such as grapes, blueberries, mulberries, plums, and apples, as well as in peanuts and pistachios
  - Curcumin: found in turmeric
  - Other polyphenols: found in grape seed, flaxseed, pumpkin seeds, and chia seeds
- **Flavonoids:** Strong antioxidants, decrease inflammation, found in several types of foods
  - Blueberries, raspberries, strawberries, cranberries, blackberries, bilberries
  - Red wine, lemons, limes, oranges, grapefruit, grapes, apples, peaches
  - Onions, broccoli, kale, lettuce, tomatoes
  - Red potatoes, red onions, radishes, plums, parsley, red peppers
  - Tea (black, oolong, green, white), rooibos, chocolate, cocoa
  - Soybeans, chickpeas, fava beans
  - Spices and herbs, including black pepper, ginger, all-spice, bay leaves, cinnamon, licorice, paprika, clove, nutmeg, chili pepper, mint, celery

This may seem like a lot to remember, but the bottom line is easy: to get a good range of phytonutrients, try to eat a rainbow of vegetables and fruits at every meal (see figure 3.4). Feel free to add tofu, chickpeas, nuts, and seeds for more anti-inflammatory and antioxidant benefits. Then enjoy a glass of unsweetened iced tea,

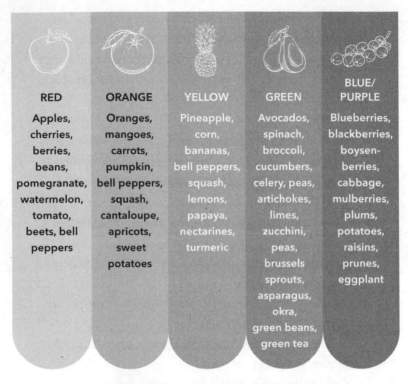

RED	ORANGE	YELLOW	GREEN	BLUE/ PURPLE
Apples, cherries, berries, beans, pomegranate, watermelon, tomato, beets, bell peppers	Oranges, mangoes, carrots, pumpkin, bell peppers, squash, cantaloupe, apricots, sweet potatoes	Pineapple, corn, bananas, bell peppers, squash, lemons, papaya, nectarines, turmeric	Avocados, spinach, broccoli, cucumbers, celery, peas, artichokes, limes, zucchini, peas, brussels sprouts, asparagus, okra, green beans, green tea	Blueberries, blackberries, boysenberries, cabbage, mulberries, plums, potatoes, raisins, prunes, eggplant

Figure 3.4. Eating the rainbow, plus some
anti-inflammatory nuts, seeds, tea, and spices,
ensures a supply of phytonutrients.

a cup of hot tea, or maybe a glass of red wine. You can finish your meal with a bowl of berries topped with mint leaves and a bite of dark chocolate. Delicious!

A note about cocoa and chocolate: Cocoa shines as a potent pain reliever, mood booster, and inflammation fighter. It has been shown to lower pain like opioids. It activates the dopamine reward system and improves mood by boosting the same neurotransmitters as antidepressants. It prevents the breakdown of natural cannabinoids to keep those feel-good vibes. Even better, it reduces IL-6, TNF-α, and other inflammatory markers. No wonder it has been called the food of the gods! But before hitting the chocolate aisle, think quality, not quantity. We need only a few ounces of dark chocolate — 70 percent or more cacao — *a week* to receive these benefits. It is important that label lists cocoa or chocolate as the first ingredient. While eating dark chocolate is one of my favorite dietary recommendations, you should indulge only after discussing your medical conditions with your physician.

Omega-3 Fatty Acids

Part of the message of the now-debunked 1992 food pyramid was to strictly limit fats. As a result, many of us have grown up with the idea that all fat is bad. But some dietary fats are important for brain and body function. In particular, substances known as omega-3 essential fatty acids act as anti-inflammatory agents, reducing levels of inflammatory cytokines, particularly TNF-α, IL-6, and CRP.

Omega-3 fatty acids and their derivatives also help build muscle. Supplementation with omega-3 fatty acids has been shown to reduce pain from osteoarthritis and rheumatoid arthritis. Analysis studies looking at inflammatory joint pain determined that omega-3 supplementation decreased pain levels, morning stiffness, the number of tender joints, and the number of NSAID pills taken. A recent study found that omega-3 fatty acid supplementation decreases spinal disc injury and slows continued degeneration. After a sports injury or muscle strain, like lifting heavy furniture, omega-3 fatty acids can aid recovery and resolve painful inflammation. Research has shown that they may also decrease muscle atrophy and enhance healing after an injury or surgery, and with aging. Omega-3 supplements with antioxidant vitamins enhance physical health, walking ability, daytime energy, and memory in older adults. This is just what we want: less medications, less pain, less inflammation, and greater well-being.

Omega-3 fatty acids have cousins known as omega-6 fatty acids. These, too, are necessary to our body functions and processes, but an excessive intake can have adverse health effects, including inflammation. The SAD has contributed to both an increase in omega-6 consumption and a decline in omega-3 consumption. This imbalance with excess omega-6 fatty acids results in more inflammation. The key is to achieve a balance.

As with phytonutrients, our bodies cannot make these essential fatty acids; we must obtain them from our diet. Eating real food is the best way to achieve an optimal balance of omega-3 and omega-6 fatty acids. The best source of omega-3 is wild, oily fish; other sources include chia seeds, walnuts, and ground flaxseed (see list below). These can be added to daily salads loaded with green leafy vegetables or sprinkled on snacks, smoothies, and home-baked foods. Keep a bag of walnuts and almonds on hand for a healthy snack.

If it's difficult for you to obtain sufficient omega-3 from the foods you eat, consider supplementation. Research studies have found that supplementing with omega-3 reduces pain and NSAID use in people with joint pain. A study looking at people with discogenic back pain found that omega-3 supplementation resulted in pain reduction for the majority of the group, and 59 percent of people were able to stop taking NSAIDs. Before starting any supplement, you must discuss it with your physician, research side effects, consider medication interactions, and find a high-quality product. The other critical step to improving our omega-6 to omega-3 ratio is to limit omega-6-rich foods.

OMEGA-3-RICH FOODS

- fatty fish and seafood, especially wild-caught salmon, mackerel, herring, tuna, trout, halibut, sardines, anchovies, and mussels

- chia seeds, ground flaxseeds, walnuts, tofu, tempeh, edamame, miso
- olive oil, butter, coconut oil, ghee
- green leafy vegetables (spinach, kale)
- brassicas (brussels sprouts, broccoli, cauliflower)
- avocados
- algae, seaweed
- hemp oil, krill oil
- enriched, free-range eggs
- grass-fed meat

OMEGA-6-RICH FOODS TO AVOID

- processed foods, especially those cooked in vegetable and corn oils, such as potato chips, fast food, packaged baked goods, deli meats
- sunflower oil and seeds, corn oil, soybean oil, cottonseed oil
- mayonnaise
- fatty meats

A Deeper Dive: Specialized Pro-resolving Mediators (SPMs)

Alpha-linolenic acid is one type of omega-3 fatty acid. It is found in flaxseed, leafy green vegetables, and other omega-3-rich plant foods. In the body, alpha-linolenic acid is converted to eicosapentaenoic acid (EPA) and docosahexaenoic acid (DHA), which produce powerful anti-inflammatory agents, including prostaglandins, leukotrienes, and specialized pro-resolving mediators (SPMs). SPMs resolve imbalances in the body. They include resolvins (which resolve inflammation), protectins (which protect the body), maresins, and lipoxins. Research has shown that SPMs reduce inflammation, reduce pain, and promote tissue healing while preventing chronic inflammation. They help heal and restore homeostasis. A study of patients with knee joint effusions found that the presence of SPMs in the knee joint fluid corresponded to less pain and lower inflammatory markers. SPMs are considered by many to be the therapy of the future to prevent chronic pain and inflammation.

Protein Sources

Proteins are the building block of our cells. We need them in order to survive, repair injuries, and grow. Daily protein requirements vary by age, gender, activity level, and other factors, but eating some protein at every meal can usually meet our protein needs and keep us full. Many of us are used to consuming animal products every day as a source of protein and other nutrients, but there are clear health benefits from following a primarily plant-based diet. Studies have demonstrated decreased levels of inflammatory markers, including CRP, in people who follow a completely plant-based diet. Plant protein meets our daily needs and helps calm painful inflammation.

This does not have to be an all-or-nothing decision. A good start is to limit the number of days each week that you consume meat and/or to limit meat consumption to one meal a day. In a sixteen-year study of over four hundred thousand people, replacing just 3 percent of animal protein with plant protein decreased death rates by 10 percent. This small dietary change packs a huge punch!

The richest sources of plant protein include legumes (beans, lentils, soy and soy products), and nuts. Some vegetables, including broccoli, green peas, spinach, asparagus, artichokes, also contain protein, as do certain seeds (particularly chia, flax, pumpkin, and hemp) and grains (quinoa, amaranth, and farro). Protein is also found in sprouted grains, spirulina, and nutritional yeast. As a bonus, plant protein usually costs less than animal protein. Swap in plant protein to lower painful inflammation, save money, and extend your healthspan.

Not all plant-based foods are created equal. As always, it is important to eat *real*, minimally processed foods. Fast-food veggie burgers and frozen meat substitutes from the grocery store are often filled with additives and other chemicals that may increase inflammation and ruin the benefits of a plant-based meal. Refined flour, soybean oil, and high-fructose corn syrup all come from plant sources — but they all feed painful inflammation. Try to avoid processed plant-based foods and stick to real, recognizable foods like those listed.

Real food does not have to be time-consuming or difficult to prepare. Nuts, vegetables, and whole fruits make delicious and easy snacks for an afternoon break, the drive home, or an after-dinner treat.

CASE STUDY

Sara, a 35-year-old, overweight woman, had suffered with muscle pain and tightness in her shoulders, neck, back, and legs since she was a teenager. The pain made it hard for her to get out of bed in morning, play with her kids, go out to dinner with friends, or do anything fun. She saw several specialists who reviewed her multiple MRIs and told her the only option was to take muscle relaxers and painkillers. When I met her, she told me she was too young to be in this much pain, and she refused to be on pills forever.

After we discussed the Relief-5R plan and how the SAD feeds painful inflammation, Sara told me that her sister had "gone vegetarian" to lose weight and help manage her allergies. At first, Sara (and her whole family) were skeptical of such a food plan. They were raised on meat and potatoes. But in two months, her sister had managed to lose some weight and lower the dose of her allergy medications.

Sara worried that a dietary change was not manageable with her work and home commitments. We fleshed out some of her concerns, including the extra time and money she thought the change would involve. We reviewed practical plant-protein swaps, easy snacks, and the importance of meal planning. Armed with the Relief-5R plan, and with nothing to lose but pain, Sara decided to try a plant-protein diet for fourteen days. She committed to planning her meals and snacks while logging her progress. She even met with a nutritionist to solidify her plan (a consultation that was covered by her insurance).

Sara was able to stick with the plan beyond the trial period she had committed to. Four weeks later, Sara felt better, was experiencing less pain and greater mobility, and had more energy to play with her kids. She found that plant protein was cheaper and quicker to prepare than animal protein. She no longer felt doomed to a life sentence of medications. Since then, Sara has continued to do well. She has modified her diet to be vegetarian four days a week and to include some animal protein on the weekends. This personalized, Relief-5R plan is helping her live a better life with less pain.

Advanced Glycation End Products (AGEs)

Advanced glycation end products (AGEs) are sugar molecules combined with proteins, nucleic acids, and lipids (fats). They are present in varying quantities in foods and are also a product of the digestive process. The body is able to process AGEs, but excessive amounts cause inflammation (marked by increased levels of CRP, TNF-α, and IL-6), oxidative stress, cell damage, and cell death. A 2021 study found that people with low back pain and lower limb pain had higher levels of AGEs. These AGEs literally *age* us, causing cellular damage and inflammation. They bind to the appropriately named receptor for advanced glycation end products (RAGE). Excess dietary AGEs increase inflammation, *rage* pain in our bodies, and are linked to obesity, which, as we have seen, is also an inflammation trigger.

Animal-based foods contain large amounts of AGEs. Processed foods intended to be stored for long periods also contain high levels of AGEs, as do foods that have undergone caramelization (including sodas) and extra browning, such as baked items, fast food, potato chips, donuts, hot dogs, deep-fried foods, and barbecued meats. This processing makes fake foods look, feel, sound, and taste like real, fresh foods even years after they are made. Sugary foods, fatty foods, and alcohol all activate RAGE and cause your body to *rage* with painful inflammation. High-temperature cooking processes, particularly frying, roasting, broiling, and grilling, create more AGEs. (This is part of the reason that my bacon-donut combination, mentioned earlier, is no good, although the protein and fat in the bacon worked to prevent the donut from spiking my blood sugar.)

A high-sugar diet, obesity, and prediabetes or diabetes also increase circulating AGEs. These sugar-coated AGE molecules are laid down in the joints, spine, brain, heart, and kidney, causing inflammation, stiffness, muscle weakness, pain, and dysfunction. This may make basic activities like getting dressed, standing, or walking painful, and prevent you from enjoying activities like hiking, golfing, traveling, or fully interacting with loved ones. Studies have shown that high dietary AGE levels cause AGE deposits in lumbar discs, resulting in stiffness and degeneration. This accelerated disc deterioration and inflammation causes low back pain.

Unprocessed, real foods such as vegetables, whole fruits, and milk have lower levels of AGEs, even after cooking. You may still enjoy high-quality, grass-fed lean meat or wild salmon, but to minimize the AGEs produced during cooking, consider the use of acidic marinades (using citrus fruits or vinegar), moist heat, shorter cooking times, or cooking at lower temperatures, such as in a slow cooker. Adding certain spices to a marinade or dry rub, as well as antioxidant plant foods, can also be beneficial (see list below).

The best way to lower inflammation is to fuel your body with raw foods and those cooked at lower temperatures: raw vegetables, fruits, unroasted nuts, legumes, tofu, yogurt, and boiled or simmered foods. Antioxidant-rich foods and polyphenols from plant foods decrease AGE formation and block RAGE. Also, low-GI index foods and lower overall calorie consumption are thought to decrease AGE-associated inflammation. Nourishing your body with a plant-based diet rich in low-GI, unprocessed food, and optional high quality, lean animal-based food builds a life with less pain and inflammation.

Low-AGE Grilling Tips
- Use an acidic marinade (lemon or lime juice, vinegar).
- Add herbs and spices such as garlic, ginger, chili pepper, thyme, turmeric, mint, and rosemary to a marinade.
- Limit meat cooking time by cutting meat into smaller pieces (and placing on skewers).
- Rotate food frequently during grilling; avoid blackening.
- Choose fish, shrimp, or lean meats.
- Remove charred areas of meat before eating.
- Include antioxidant foods, such as bell peppers, onions, zucchini, and pineapple.

Hydration

Our focus has been on food. What about drinks? Dehydration is a pain assault. Studies using functional MRIs of the brain have shown that dehydration spikes pain activity and lowers our pain threshold. In other words, we feel more pain and feel it more easily. Not staying hydrated is like taking pills to cause more pain.

Water allows our cells to function. While people may think hydration mainly affects the kidneys, blood vessels, and heart, it also plays a vital role in orthopaedic health. Water hydrates our joints and spinal discs. Muscle strength and performance depend on a proper balance of water and electrolytes. Studies have shown that dehydration also affects brain function and mood, contributes to constipation, and shifts our bodies to a high-inflammation state. Less water means that less oxygen and fewer nutrients are delivered to our spine and joints. In other words, when our bodies are not adequately hydrated, fewer anti-inflammatory, healing, and regenerative molecules are circulating to heal and prevent back, joint, and muscle pain.

Water is essential, but other drinks contain compounds that can help crush inflammation and provide important nutrients. Green tea and black tea contain powerful antioxidants; like ninja warriors, they defend the body and slash inflammation. Green tea also decreases inflammatory markers, protects cartilage, and prevents muscle atrophy. Tea helps reduce pain related to arthritis, joint degeneration, muscle pain, and spine pain. Other drinks, including various types of milk, are potential sources of calcium, vitamin D, and protein.

We already know that we should avoid sugary drinks if we want to reduce painful inflammation. Alcohol dehydrates the body in addition to causing other forms of damage. Limiting our intake benefits us in numerous ways.

Try to make water your go-to drink. If that sounds bland, it helps to add a slice of lime, lemon, or cucumber to your glass; or try sparkling water with no sweeteners. Some ways to increase your water intake include drinking a glass each morning after you brush your teeth, before every snack, and before every meal. Your joints, muscles, and spine will thank you!

Intolerances and Sensitivities

A food *intolerance* occurs when a person does not have a nutrient or enzyme necessary to break down or metabolize the food. This triggers discomfort and inflammation. A food *sensitivity* occurs when the body reacts to a food and symptoms appear several hours or days later. These are different from food *allergies*, which are more immediate immune responses characterized by hives, itchiness, swelling, and anaphylaxis. Because of their quick onset and distinct symptoms and signs, food allergies are the more obvious. Many people may not even know that they suffer from food intolerances and sensitivities, yet both can contribute to ongoing musculoskeletal pain and a multitude of other symptoms.

COMMON TRIGGERS OF INTOLERANCE AND SENSITIVITY
- **Food intolerance**
  - dairy products
  - histamine-rich foods such as deli meats, alcohol, aged cheese, citrus fruits
  - artificial flavors and coloring
  - preservatives
- **Food sensitivity**
  - dairy products
  - eggs
  - gluten
  - soy
  - shellfish
  - tree nuts

If you suspect certain foods may be triggering inflammation, consider temporarily eliminating the "usual suspects" from your diet. The big three are dairy products, gluten, and alcohol. The traditional approach to identifying triggers eliminates all possible triggers from the diet and reintroduces them gradually, one at a time. If you are considering an elimination diet, it is best to meet with a specialized physician and nutritionist for guidance.

A less drastic approach is to eliminate a single food or food group from your diet and see whether you feel better. Drinking no alcohol for four weeks has no nutritional downside and will readily reveal whether alcohol contributes to your pain and dysfunction. If you are considering eliminating gluten or dairy products, be sure you are getting necessary nutrients from alternative sources.

CASE STUDY

Drew, an active 28-year-old man, threw his back out while shoveling snow. The severe pain resolved in a few weeks, but a nagging low back pain lingered. Anytime he tried to run, lift weights, or even play basketball, his entire back would freeze, leaving him unable to stand up straight. Physical therapy and NSAIDs provided only limited relief. As an expectant father, Drew worried that he would not be able to be the hands-on dad he wanted to be.

Drew was diagnosed with disc degeneration, disc herniation, and spasms. Because he did not have leg pain, he was not considered a candidate for surgery. He felt stuck. When he met with me, we discussed conventional treatments, from prescription medications to epidural steroid injections. He made it clear that he wanted to eliminate the cause of the pain, not cover it up with a Band-aid treatment.

I introduced Drew to the Relief-5R plan. While he did not have problems with exercise, sleep, or stress (addressed by the Revitalize, Recharge, and Refresh pillars of the program), we discovered food was a big factor. In his family, he was known as the human garbage disposal.

Because he could (and did) eat anything and everything without gaining weight, he had never worried about his eating habits. We discussed SAD, inflammatory foods, and elimination diets. He decided to try a two-week elimination diet – no dairy, no meat, and no alcohol. In three days, his back pain had diminished. In four weeks, he had resumed playing basketball with his friends. More than a year later, he continues with better food choices because he feels better. On the weekends, he drinks alcohol socially, but he has no desire to return to eating dairy products or animal protein. His wife has adopted the same diet, and they both enjoy the benefits of freedom from long-term pain medications. He is free of his back pain, enjoying an active life, and becoming the father he dreamed of being.

The Gut Microbiome

Our digestive tract is populated by more than a trillion tiny organisms, including bacteria, viruses, fungi, and yeast that are together called the gut microbiome. They help us, and we help them. Spoiler alert: they affect pain and inflammation levels! An optimal microbiome helps us digest food, absorb vitamins, fight infections, and lower painful inflammation. An unbalanced gut microbiome causes chaos, dysfunction, and pain.

Poor diet, infections, stress, surgery, and certain medications can wipe out some beneficial gut organisms and enable the growth of harmful ones. Studies have found that an unbalanced gut microbiome correlates with chronic musculoskeletal pain. The SAD directly affects the "gut-joint axis" and leads to more swelling, more inflammation, more pain, and more dysfunction.

Certain foods support a healthy microbiome and feed the

beneficial bacteria. These types of foods are called *prebiotics*. They include foods high in fiber and low in sugar. Some excellent prebiotic foods are onions, apples, asparagus, artichokes, cabbage, almonds, leeks, flaxseeds, seaweed, and leafy greens. We can also maintain a healthy gut biome by eating foods that contain beneficial bacteria. These foods, known as *probiotics*, include cultured and fermented foods such as plain, unsweetened yogurt, kimchi, sauerkraut, pickles, miso, and tempeh. The bottom line is to focus on vegetables, high-fiber fruits, unprocessed foods, and fermented foods for a balanced microbiome.

Any oral medication can disrupt the gut microbiome, but some are notorious for this, including NSAIDs and antibiotics. NSAIDs change the gut microbiome composition, block the production of gut-protective substances, and can injure the gut lining. All these effects lead to dysbiosis, a gut microbiome imbalance. While antibiotics can be life-saving, it is important to use them only as prescribed by a physician to treat a bacterial infection. As their name suggests, *anti*-biotics do not discriminate between harmful and helpful bacteria (biotics): they often wipe out the good guys right along with the bad guys. When beginning a course of antibiotics, it is important to discuss this possible adverse effect with your physician. Together, you may decide to increase your consumption of prebiotic and/or probiotic foods to keep your gut balanced. Avoiding processed foods, inactivity, and stress (more in chapter 6, "Refresh") helps promote a happy, healthy microbiome.

MAINTAINING A HEALTHY GUT MICROBIOME
- Keep hydrated.
- Eat high-fiber foods.
- Eat fermented foods.

- Avoid foods with added sugar and artificial ingredients.
- Limit stress.
- Avoid long-term use of NSAIDs.
- Stay physically active.

Supplements

The best way to decrease painful inflammation is to eat real food. Period. However, some people may benefit from nutritional supplements to fill dietary deficiencies (such as those resulting from food insensitivities or intolerances). Supplements, like medications, have side effects and may interact with medications, other supplements, and vitamins. Several supplements are known to cause an increased risk of bleeding, nausea, vomiting, and diarrhea. Supplements may have unreported side effects as well. Therefore, all supplements must be discussed with your physician.

Below is list of a few potentially helpful supplements for reducing painful inflammation. Studies have found that these supplements exert anti-inflammatory and antioxidant effects. Some temper the inflammation cascade, like NSAIDs, but without blocking the production of beneficial substances.

- Nutritional and oral supplements
  - turmeric
  - boswellia
  - bromelain
  - ginger
  - quercetin
  - green tea
  - black tea
  - specialized pro-resolving mediators (SPMs)

- omega-3 fatty acids (DHA/EPA)
- licorice root
- milk thistle
- resveratrol
- Chinese skullcap
- cat's claw
- melatonin
- vitamins, including C and D

The Role of Spices

One way to enhance the benefits of a plant-based, nutrient-dense diet is to add spices with anti-inflammatory properties, such as those listed below. Studies have found that these spices reduce inflammatory cytokines.

Anti-Inflammatory Powerhouse Spices and Herbs

turmeric	oregano
ginger	cocoa powder
garlic	rosemary
pepper	basil
cloves	thyme
peppermint	

Sprinkle these powerhouse spices on raw vegetables, fruits, and cooked dishes. These tiny boosts help soothe chronic inflammation, arthritic dysfunction, and musculoskeletal pain.

Fasting

We've talked about how to eat; what about how *not* to eat? There is evidence that intermittent fasting — a catchall term for calorie restriction over a defined period — may aid in controlling pain and inflammation. People fasting for religious reasons exhibit lower levels of inflammatory substances (including TNF-α, IL-6, and CRP) compared to nonfasting control groups. Furthermore, studies have also shown that periodic fasting reduces arthritic pain and inflammation. A 2020 study discovered that intermittent fasting increases sensitivity to opioid pain medications and reduces the amount of medication needed. This translates to less pain with fewer opioids, NSAIDs, invasive procedures, or expensive endeavors. A review of multiple studies on people with fibromyalgia, a painful musculoskeletal condition, found that a lower-calorie diet reduced pain and increased function. It also reduced anxiety, depression, and inflammatory markers, and improved sleep quality and quality of life. As a bonus, intermittent fasting improves healthspan, cellular function, and blood-sugar control.

Fasting reduces painful inflammation through multiple mechanisms. Weight loss may be a factor, but it is not the main mechanism. More important, fasting reduces the time and energy our bodies spend repeatedly processing food, removing toxins, and balancing our blood sugars. It is exhausting even thinking about the cycle of digestion. Our bodies may have just finished metabolizing a meal and recovering from a blood-sugar spike when we reach for our mid-morning, afternoon, or bedtime snack and restart the whole process! Human bodies are not designed for eating this frequently. Our ancestors did not have constant access to pantries full of food, convenience stores, and indulgent snacks. Our bodies need a break from constant food input just like our minds need a break from constant social media input.

Often, intermittent fasting results in less calorie consumption.

This has been shown time and again to improve health and reduce inflammation. Fasting and calorie restriction both activate autophagy, which is a fancy word for cleaning up, recycling, and removing cellular garbage (including inflammatory substances). If we give the body a break from constant food processing, it can remove inflammatory substances more effectively.

Autophagy and painful inflammation share a deeper, spookier connection. As part of autophagy, the immune system cleans out old, damaged cells, making way for new cells to develop. Sometimes, these damaged cells refuse to die and instead continuously pump out inflammatory substances. These "zombie cells" poison everything around them like a rotten apple. They spike inflammation, which results in more joint, back, and muscle pain. Studies have shown that intermittent fasting suppresses this cellular activity, preventing a zombie-cell apocalypse.

Intermittent fasting must be discussed with your physician first, particularly if you have blood sugar problems, blood pressure problems, heart conditions, hormone conditions, or eating disorders, or if you are pregnant or breastfeeding.

BENEFITS OF INTERMITTENT FASTING
- reduced pain
- reduced inflammation
- reduced inflammatory fat
- reduced metabolic syndrome risk factors
- lowered cholesterol
- increased levels of antioxidants
- improved blood sugar control
- improved stress resistance
- improved endurance, balance, and coordination
- lowered blood pressure

- improved brain function (cognition, memory, learning)
- improved emotional well-being

Types of Fasting

There are several popular approaches to fasting that work to suit people with different needs and lifestyles. A good way to think of it is not as going hungry but rather as defining our eating periods. These do not have to be unrealistic, hard lines but simply guidelines. For example, restricting our eating to the hours between 7 a.m. and 7 p.m. is not a drastic limitation but is more beneficial than an eating period that extends late into the night. With a twelve-hour eating period, you are unlikely to feel hungry or weak if you have been cleared to try this eating pattern by your personal physician.

- **Daily time-restricted:** Eating only during limited hours each day: for example, between 9 a.m. and 6 p.m.
- **Modified fasting:** Restricting intake for a certain number of days each week: for example, eating no more than six hundred calories a day on Monday and Thursday. Fasting for two out of seven days each week is known as 5:2 fasting.
- **Alternate-day fasting:** Restricting or avoiding eating every other day.

On intense fasting days, you must monitor how you feel, avoid rigorous exercise, and stay well hydrated. Once again, these eating patterns should only be attempted if cleared by your physician. The concept is to focus on real, unprocessed foods with the most nutrition in the lowest number of calories. You still need to ensure that you get a healthy intake of vitamins, minerals, fats, and proteins. A nutritionist can help design an optimal plan.

Circadian Eating

Many people consistently find that their pain worsens at certain times of the day. Our circadian rhythm — our internal clock — regulates our sleep-wake cycle and is affected by light levels. It influences the levels of various hormones, including stress hormones, hunger hormones, and sleep hormones, and these in turn affect our experience of pain. A 2021 article reviewed the complex relationship between circadian rhythm and chronic pain and showed that neuroinflammation is related to melatonin and light exposure. We can tailor treatments around these circadian patterns. It is also important to recognize that most pain is worse with sleep deprivation (more on this in chapter 5, "Recharge").

If we work in sync with our circadian rhythm, we can function better, with less inflammation and pain. Circadian eating and circadian fasting are natural ways to lower pain, inflammation, and dysfunction.

POTENTIAL BENEFITS OF CIRCADIAN EATING

- less pain
- less inflammation
- better gut health
- lower risk of metabolic diseases
- better sleep
- better weight control

If you are cleared by your medical team to practice intermittent fasting, try scheduling it in sync with your circadian rhythm, so that you eat mainly during daylight hours. For a simple start, try eating from 7 a.m. to 7 p.m. only. If you are practicing ten-hour time-restricted fasting, set your schedule so that you eat between 8 a.m. and 6 p.m. instead of between 11 a.m. and 9 p.m. Research studies show that early time-restricted eating results in less inflammation, better blood sugar control, and better food metabolism compared to later time-restricted eating, and may increase autophagy.

Low-Inflammation Fuel

How do we use food to program our bodies for less pain? We know the SAD results in more inflammation, pain, and *dis*-ease. A diet of unprocessed foods, low-GI, and high-fiber foods, especially vegetables and fruits, helps reduce pain, restore gut balance, and decrease inflammation. A randomized controlled study reported in *Pain Medicine* found that adopting a low-carbohydrate diet (with leafy green vegetables and non-starchy vegetables) resulted in less pain, less inflammation, less oxidative stress, and more function in only twelve weeks. The authors suggested that dietary improvements might be a way to reduce opioid and other medication use. Real food can help minimize our need for dangerous medications and lower the risks of organ damage, addiction, and death. Ready to start?

A Mediterranean-style diet has been found in multiple studies to decrease pain and disability for people with joint pain. This type of diet, incorporating lots of fresh vegetables, fish and seafood, and small servings of lean meat, shifts your body to ease, relief, and wellness. While there are many complicated ways to upgrade your fuel, and diets tailored to the relief of particular conditions (including an anti-inflammatory diet for arthritis sufferers), the easiest and most sustainable way is a shift from processed food to real food. Adhering to a few guiding principles works better than obsessing over calorie counts, micronutrients, and grams of carbohydrates. You can use these principles to plan your meals for the week ahead and batch cook on the weekend. This can be a fun, music-filled, or group activity to save time during the busy work week and prevent last-minute reaches for inflammatory, processed foods.

GUIDE TO LOW-INFLAMMATORY EATING

- Eat and cook with real (one-ingredient) foods as much as possible.
- Avoid processed foods.
- Reduce your intake of foods with added sugars, added salt, or artificial additives (sweeteners, flavors, colors).
- Eat a rainbow of plant-based foods to obtain healthy phytonutrients.
- Consume natural, prebiotic, high-fiber foods.
- Include nuts, legumes, healthy seeds, and anti-inflammatory spices in your snacks and meals.
- Look for low-GI foods.
- Choose drinks with no added sweeteners.
- Cook foods with healthy, omega-3 oils and in ways that minimize AGE formation.
- Consider replacing meat with beans and legumes two or three days a week.
- Choose fatty fishes, like wild-caught salmon in lieu of meat.
- Choose whole-grain cereals, breads, and pasta.

My five favorite pain-fighting superfoods are berries, fatty fish, colorful vegetables, green tea, and powerhouse spices. Focus on all the wonderful, beneficial, pain-relieving foods you can enjoy.

A FOOD PLAN TO LOWER INFLAMMATION

1. Think about your goals.
2. Try to include more of the following in your diet:
   - real food
   - phytonutrient-rich, colorful food
   - omega-3 fatty acids from sources such as fatty fishes and omega-3 rich oils
   - fiber
   - plant-based proteins: legumes, nuts, seeds

- anti-inflammatory spices and herbs
- low-GI foods
- prebiotic and probiotic foods
- water
- unsweetened tea

3. Try to reduce or avoid the following items:
   - processed foods
   - added sugar
   - high-AGE foods or cooking methods
   - excess omega-6 fatty acids
   - low-fiber foods
   - high-GI foods
   - animal fat
   - alcohol
4. Consider an elimination trial of dairy and gluten.
5. Make some notes about how to make this plan work for you.
6. Bon appetit!

It can be difficult to eliminate some foods and ingredients that we are used to consuming. Table 3.1 contains some convenient and tasty substitutes for inflammatory foods.

Table 3.1. Fuel for reducing pain and inflammation.

INSTEAD OF...	TRY...
Soda, juice, diet soda, alcohol	Water, sparkling water, tea
Processed, high-AGE snacks (potato chips, tortilla chips)	Crunchy vegetables (with hummus, salsa, or guacamole), nuts, seeds, fruit
High-fat meat, processed meats	Fish, beans, legumes, tofu, high-quality lean and grass-fed meat

INSTEAD OF ...	TRY ...
Candy, cookies	Peanut butter, almond butter, homemade energy bites, fruit, homemade cookies, plain yogurt with berries, dark chocolate
Vegetable, peanut, and sunflower oils, margarine	Butter, ghee, extra-virgin olive oil; sesame, walnut, almond, flaxseed, and avocado oils

The Bottom Line

Fuel can feed or quell painful inflammation (figure 3.5). The choice is up to us. The ideal fuel allows us to feel better and achieve our goals.

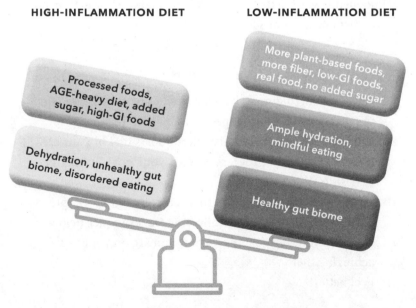

Figure 3.5. Refuel plan for orthopaedic
ease and wellness.

Refuel Microboosts

The mnemonic *RELIEF* can help you find easy ways to add microboosts to your day (figure 3.6). Think of it like setting up a store — keep all the things you want to focus on at eye level and attractively displayed. Use "I" declarations to state and write your plan — this helps make microboosts stick and helps you commit to them. Together these steps make it easier for you to accomplish your microboosts and feel better.

There will always be setbacks. Be prepared for them by having a plan to start afresh the next day. An occasional sugary indulgence or fast-food meal is not a failure, as long as it does not become a pattern. To get back on track, look at your big goals and microboosts. Think about tweaks that might make your plan more successful, and start again, reviewing your plan daily.

Rewards drive success. Celebrate your wins (big and small), acknowledge your setbacks, and keep moving forward for more pain relief and a better life.

Next Steps

1. Review your big goal — what you want to achieve (or prevent) by making changes.
2. From the list below, identify microboosts that fit your life and will help you progress toward your goal. It may be easiest to start with two.
3. Turn these microboosts into a custom Relief-5R plan with specific action steps, following the examples below.
4. Envision your big goals and know you are on your way to achieving them
5. Feel better!

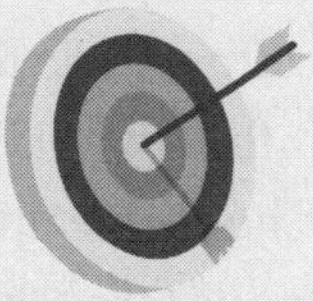

SET FOR SUCCESS: REFUEL

R REMOVE BARRIERS
- **Intention:** Eat healthier snacks.
- **Microboost:** *I will keep nuts in the front of the pantry and ditch processed snacks.*

E EYE LEVEL
- **Intention:** Drink more water.
- **Microboost:** *Each night, I will fill a reusable water bottle and put it in the front of the fridge.*

L LINK TO A SPECIFIC ACTIVITY
- **Intention:** Eat more plant-based foods.
- **Microboost:** *At dinner, I will fill half my plate with vegetables.*

I "I" DECLARATION
- **Intention:** Eat more fruit.
- **Microboost:** *I will say aloud, "I like eating berries." I will write down, "I will eat berries for dessert."*

E ENCOURAGE PROGRESS BY TRACKING
- **Intention:** Keep track of my progress.
- **Microboost:** *I will use a calendar or app to track each daily accomplishment.*

F FEEL BETTER!

Figure 3.6. Relief-5R method for creating customized Refuel microboosts.

MICROBOOSTS: LEVEL 1
- Increase your intake of inflammation-fighting fruit, nuts, colorful vegetables, whole grains, and omega-3 fatty acids.
- Load your fridge and freezer with veggies and fruits.
- Eat real, recognizable foods.

- Plan a week's worth of meals to reduce the burden of deciding what to eat and the temptation to turn to quick, inflammatory foods.
- Choose healthy substitutes for inflammatory, processed foods (see table 3.1, pp. 76–77).
- Add the five superfoods to your diet: berries, colorful vegetables, fatty fish, green tea, and powerhouse spices and herbs.
- Read product labels and avoid added salt, sugar (in all its forms), and artificial ingredients.
- Replace animal protein with plant protein at least one day a week.
- Make sure each meal or snack contains some protein, fiber, and fats rich in omega-3 fatty acid. This prevents you from feeling hangry and eliminates mid-morning and late-afternoon slumps.
- Skip the snack aisle at the grocery store.
- Stock your kitchen with nutritious, anti-inflammatory snacks, such as guacamole, hummus, salsa, veggies, fruits, nuts, and nut butters.
- For snacking on the go, pack up some sliced vegetables, a bag of nuts, and almond butter or hummus with whole-grain crackers.
- Increase the amount of water you drink.
- Replace soda, diet soda, sports drinks, juices, sweetened coffee, and sweetened tea with plain water, sparkling water, and unsweetened iced tea, tea, or coffee.
- If you drink alcohol, try going alcohol-free for a month. Record your energy, activity, and pain levels daily and see whether you notice improvement.

Microboosts Level 2 (Advanced)

- Try eating no processed food for fourteen days. Record your energy, activity, and pain levels daily and see whether you notice improvement.
- Replace animal protein with plant protein four or five days a week.
- If your physician agrees, consider circadian and time-restricted fasting.
- If you think you may have a food intolerance or sensitivity, discuss doing an elimination diet with your physician.

Custom Relief Plan: Examples

- *I will fill half of my plate with vegetables at dinner.*
- *I will check product labels for added sugar at the grocery store and buy less of these products.*
- *I will switch my after-dinner dessert from a processed food to fruit.*
- *I will fill my water bottle for the next day and put it in the fridge right before bedtime.*
- *I will pack "real fast food" (nuts, hummus, guacamole, trail mix) for a snack.*
- *I will replace animal protein with less-inflammatory plant protein every Thursday.*
- *I will track my progress at bedtime with stickers and a calendar.*

CHAPTER 4

Revitalize

*Movement offers us pleasure, identity, belonging and hope.
It puts us in places that are good for us, whether that's
outdoors in nature, in an environment that challenges us,
or with a supportive community.*

— Kelly McGonigal

Myth: To relieve orthopaedic pain, we should avoid
physical activity.
Fact: Inactivity worsens chronic orthopaedic pain and
inflammation.
Relief-5R: Revitalizing with more movement is part
of a true pain solution.

When most people think about relieving orthopaedic pain,
they think about rest, medications, physical therapy, and
surgery. Most people focus on treating the specific body area
causing pain. While this approach is appropriate following an
acute injury, for ongoing pain reduction and pain prevention, we

need to get moving. The pain-relieving benefits of exercise extend beyond stretching and strengthening the affected area; movement helps the whole person, body and mind. And it doesn't require paying a fee to work out at a gym! Integrating more activity and movement into your daily routine can prevent pain, release stress, lower inflammation, and extend your healthspan.

The Benefits of Movement

Many years ago, doctors recommended bed rest for orthopaedic pain and injuries. Today we know better. Inactivity weakens our muscles, joints, and bones. Immobility reduces blood flow and thus the supply of nutrients to the injured area. This supports the old rehab saying "Use it or lose it." As long as your physician confirms that there is no instability, fracture, or danger in moving, movement promotes healing, pain relief, and wellness.

If there were a vitamin or pill to prevent future chronic pain, would you take it? Most people gladly would. Yet a preventive already exists: more daily movement. It prevents diffuse, nagging, ongoing pain and benefits us in a multitude of other ways. A study spanning more than a decade found that people who exercised regularly had less chronic musculoskeletal pain and widespread pain. *Exercise protects against pain.*

Inactivity and prolonged sitting are well-established risk factors for low back pain. The more physically inactive a person is, the more likely they are to have compressed lumbar discs, fatty atrophy of the spinal muscles, increased back pain, and some degree of disability. Prolonged sitting is associated with biochemical markers of chronic, ongoing inflammation — just like eating processed foods. A 2020 study found that more time spent sitting correlated with higher rates of inflammatory diseases like heart disease, metabolic disease, and diabetes. Even worse, a study published in the *Journal of the American Medical Association* found that greater time spent sitting correlates with a greater risk of dying from cancer. Inactivity and prolonged sitting not only worsen pain but may shorten our lives. The antidote is movement.

Benefits of Movement

- less inflammation
- less pain
- lower risk of repetitive muscle strain
- improved sleep
- improved circulation
- improved bone health
- increased calorie use
- improved muscle tone
- lower blood sugar
- extended lifespan and healthspan
- lower risk of heart disease and cancer
- lower stress
- better mental focus

Movement pumps up immune function and improves mind-body function. Scientists have dubbed it *neuroprotective*, meaning that it protects the brain and prevents nerve cell death. With a healthier brain, we can make better decisions to cope with and eliminate pain.

In addition, exercise itself can reduce chronic pain. Whole-body exercise, like walking, biking, or dancing, can help reduce pain in specific parts of the body. Seated exercises that use the large muscles, like chair yoga and seated tai chi, can also be helpful. This physiological response to movement is known as *exercise-induced hypoalgesia*.

Since movement leads to better sleep, healthier eating habits, less stress, and reduced feelings of loneliness, all of which are interrelated, it supports the other pillars of the Relief-5R plan.

If all this is true, why doesn't everybody love exercise? Sometimes it seems daunting to add formal exercise to our day. Spending an hour a day at the gym may be unrealistic given limited time, pain levels, lack of endurance, transportation difficulties, or other factors. But more movement does not mean dedicating a big chunk of time to exercise. Little microboosts of movement throughout the day add up to big relief.

Sometimes the benefits of making little changes do not inspire action. In weighing our choices, we need to keep in mind that inactivity results in muscle atrophy, more inflammation, poor sleep, poor food choices, and more chronic pain (figure 4.1). More movement may save us from muscle wasting, falls, injury, and pain down the road.

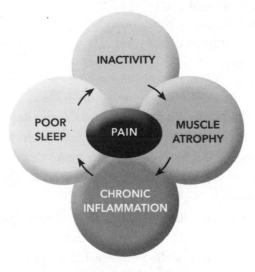

Figure 4.1. The cycle of inactivity.

Exercise as a Natural Painkiller

Movement, activity, and less sitting trigger natural pain relievers in our body and brain. A 2020 analysis of fifteen studies on people with pain found that exercise increases pain tolerance and reduces pain sensitivity more than massage, pain education, and stress-management techniques. Movement not only improves and strengthens our pain-fighting muscles; it also leads to the release of various chemicals in the body that reduce pain, lower inflammation, and leave us feeling good. Here's the breakdown of this pain-relief sauce.

Endorphins

Have you heard of an "exercise high"? It is real. Our bodies produce hormones known as endorphins that function like natural opioids: they decrease pain and make us feel good. This feeling of well-being encourages us to exercise more. Naturally released endorphins are safer, better alternatives to narcotics and other dangerous medications. Scientists are even trying to bottle the benefits of exercise into medications called *exercise mimetics*.

Vigorous aerobic exercise triggers the biggest release of endorphins, but it's not only elite athletes who benefit from an exercise high. Moderate-intensity exercise decreases pain. What's more, the exercise does not have to target the injured or painful area. A recent study found that leg exercises can decrease shoulder pain! So even if part of your body feels too tender or inflamed to exercise, consider gentle movement or exercise that targets other parts of your body to release pain-fighting endorphins.

Endocannabinoids

Medical marijuana (cannabis) has been shown to help reduce pain. The fact that our bodies respond to marijuana in this way makes sense when we consider that they produce their own cannabis-like substances, called endocannabinoids, that relieve pain. One of these endocannabinoids is the aptly named anandamide, from the Sanskrit word *ananda*, meaning "bliss."

So how do you experience some *ananda*? Through movement.

Studies have found that moderately intense activity on a stationary bike activates the production of endocannabinoids, reducing pain, lowering anxiety, and creating a sense of well-being.

Serotonin

Exercise increases levels of serotonin, a neurotransmitter that contributes to pain relief. Serotonin is also implicated in healing, mood, bone health, appetite regulation, and sleep. Interestingly, the most commonly prescribed antidepressants are selective serotonin reuptake inhibitors (SSRIs), which work by increasing the amount of serotonin circulating in the brain. Exercise does it for free, without medication side effects.

Myokines

Beyond releasing natural pain relievers and mood boosters, increased activity lowers inflammation. When muscles contract, they produce myokines, cell messengers that reduce acute inflammation and chronic inflammation. They also influence mood and learning ability. Myokines help prevent muscle wasting, obesity, and early aging. These homemade anti-inflammatories fight painful inflammation with a few, frequent clicks of your heels. This is why researchers recommend exercise as an anti-inflammatory treatment for painful arthritic conditions.

Numerous studies have demonstrated the anti-inflammatory benefits of exercise. In a study of overweight and obese people, regular, moderate-intensity walking resulted in less inflammation (as measured by levels of TNF-α) in only four weeks. Another study found that just twenty minutes of moderate walking lowered inflammation (measured by TNF-α levels) acutely. Walking at moderate intensity for twenty to thirty minutes a day can lower inflammation and reduce the need for pain medication. Exercise decreases whole-body inflammation, inflammatory fat, and oxidative stress that contribute to more pain, disability, and systemic conditions like heart disease and stroke. More movement is win-win-win-win.

Getting in Gear

The best way to move more is to incorporate fun, interactive, and outdoor exercise into your life; this could be walking, dancing, hiking, biking, swimming, or seated yoga. Outdoor activities and activities enjoyed with a friend or family member are a double win because both being outdoors and positive social interactions also reduce pain, inflammation, and dysfunction. As part of the Relief-5R plan, we lower pain by investing in ourselves. This shift begins with boosting our food choices and activity level to feel better.

Our society promotes a "work hard, play hard" and an all-or-nothing attitude. This can deter people who think an exercise program inevitably requires a gym membership, hours of time, and suffering. Relief lies in moderation. Moderate-intensity activities are those that raise your heart rate and breathing rate to a degree that allows you to carry on a conversation, but not to sing, such as those listed below. It is important to start at your own pace and work up to these goals once you have been cleared for an exercise program by your physician.

- brisk walking (at a pace of more than 3 miles per hour)
- bicycling (10–12 miles per hour)
- swimming
- recreational dancing
- vacuuming
- mopping
- playing badminton
- playing tennis doubles

Many of us sit for the majority of the day at work or at home, to say nothing of the commute. We sit at dinner. Then we follow up with a big serving of sitting to watch TV, surf the internet, or read. Prolonged sitting hurts us in the long run, yet our lives seem centered on it.

We need to intentionally break up our seated activities. This may mean buying or making an adjustable sitting/standing desk. It may mean setting a phone alarm to stretch every hour, like my brother, a computer engineer. It may mean taking an extra walk to the bathroom, kitchen, or break room in the morning and afternoon. It may mean walking during phone meetings. It boils down to inserting little bits of standing or activity to your day. Those at home can create a "fake commute." This means taking a morning walk around your neighborhood to signal the start of the work day and another walk to demarcate the end of the work day. The "fake commute" adds more movement to your day and helps set boundaries between work and home life.

Experts recommend thirty minutes of dedicated physical activity a day. But half an hour of movement does not compensate for 23.5 hours of inactivity. Even if you work out daily, small bursts of movement, position changes, and stretches throughout the day help lower stress, inflammation, and pain.

Have you heard the recommendation to walk ten thousand steps a day? There is some merit to this idea, but like any lifestyle change, it has to work in your world if you are going to stick with it. For some people, ten thousand steps may be an unrealistic or inappropriate goal. A study published in the *Journal of the American Medical Association* found that lifespan increased in women walking 4,400 steps or more a day.

Whether counting steps, going to the gym, hiking with a friend, dancing, practicing yoga, or completing mini-exercise routines, adding more movement to our day relieves pain and improves well-being (figure 4.2). And no matter what your exercise goals may be, keeping track of your progress can be a great motivator. Studies have shown that using a smartphone or other exercise tracking device increases physical activity by giving us daily gratification and the daily confirmation that "we got our steps in."

ACTIVITIES

Biking, hiking, jogging, swimming, tennis, karate, jumping rope, rock climbing, dancing, skiing, and other sports.

GET A SITTING/ STANDING DESK

Buy or make one, and alternate between sitting and standing. An antifatigue floor mat may increase standing comfort.

DAILY WALK

Set a time for a daily walk — maybe first thing in the morning or after dinner every day. If the weather is poor, substitute an online exercise video or yoga.

MOVE ALARM

Set an alarm on your watch, phone, or computer to remind you to get up and stretch or to switch from sitting to standing.

PARK AND WALK

Park farther away and walk more at work, restaurants, and stores.

INVEST IN YOU

Your wellness matters. It allows you to function and take care of others. Make time to care for yourself and feel better.

USE THE STAIRS

Enough said.

Figure 4.2. More than steps: ways to move more and move more often.

Sometimes it helps to have additional forms of motivation, such as an exercise partner or group, a good instructor, an attractive setting, or a great workout playlist. A 2021 study found that medium-tempo music improved enjoyment, perceived exertion, and remembered pleasure. The right music helps us feel better during and after exercise. It locks in a good memory that motivates us to repeat the experience.

Movement breaks are even better with a partner or group. Active socializing helps reduce pain, inflammation, and stress (more on this in chapter 7, "Relate"), so socializing while you exercise is a double win! It also keeps you accountable on days when you might be tempted to skip a solitary walk or workout. Some people enjoy meeting a friend for a hike or a walk around the mall before it opens. Others prefer going to a dance or yoga class, or playing tennis or basketball with friends. For me, simplicity reigns supreme. I enjoy a daily evening walk with my family, by myself in nature, or while talking on the phone to a loved one.

Mix up where you walk and who you exercise with, in person or on the phone. Taking a brief lunchtime walk with a work friend adds more movement and supportive social connection to your day. Even if your current pain levels or daily schedules allow for only ten- or fifteen-minute chunks of walking, they still count: go for it on a work break, while watching your child's soccer practice, or after dinner. If you are stuck indoors, develop a go-to, hourly stretching routine to break up prolonged time in any one position. It may be as simple as neck rolls and shoulder shrugs, or it could include some of the following movements in a sturdy chair if cleared by your physician.

- **Five-minute walk**
- **Arm circles:** Stand with arms extended and move them in small circles in each direction.
- **Back stretches:** Follow the recommendations of a physical therapist.

- **Calf lifts:** Hold your desk or chair for support while alternating between standing on your toes and flat on your feet.
- **Chair sit to stand:** With your feet flat on the floor, try to stand up without using your arms and hands, or using them as little as possible.
- **Chair squats:** Standing in front of a stable chair, bend or cross your arms, and squat down to just above the level of the chair seat.
- **Desk pushups:** If your desk is sturdy, stand up, step back from your desk, and lean your hands on the edge of the desk. With your feet flat on the ground and back straight, do a pushup. If this is too difficult or your desk is not sturdy, consider wall pushups, described below.
- **Knee to chest:** Seated on a stable chair with your back pressed against the chair back, keep one foot on the ground, and hug the other knee toward your chest. Repeat with the other leg.
- **Leg extensions:** While seated, keep one foot on the floor, tighten your abdominal muscles, and raise and extend the other foot until your leg is straight. Repeat with the other leg.
- **Lunges**
- **Neck, shoulder, wrist, and ankle rolls**
- **Reach for the sky:** Hold your hands up and reach for the sky.
- **Resistance band exercises:** Follow the recommendations of a physical therapist.
- **Wall pushups:** Stand a couple of feet away from the wall and place your hands flat on the wall, wider than your shoulders. Keeping your back straight, do a pushup against the wall. For a greater challenge, stand farther away from the wall.

- **Wall sits:** With your back against a wall, assume a seated position, with your hips and knees at ninety-degree angles. Try to hold for ten to twenty seconds.

Ergonomics

In between activity breaks, we can enhance our musculoskeletal well-being and reduce pain by being mindful of ergonomics. Good ergonomics means maintaining proper posture, good joint alignment, and a comfortable body position while performing repetitive or strenuous activities. This matters at home and at work. The recent rise in home computer use, from working at home to video meetings with friends and family, has led to a high incidence of back and neck pain. Good ergonomics and frequent movement can prevent it.

When lifting heavy objects, at work or home, being mindful can prevent an injury. A soft back brace (made of fabric and elastic) may be beneficial for repetitive heavy lifting. It provides a gentle reminder to keep good form. Unless your job requires continuous lifting, limit soft brace use to one or two hours a day so that you do not weaken your core muscles. If you need to turn around while carrying a heavy object, avoid twisting while lifting, as this can hurt your back and joints. It is better to lift, keep the item close to your core, and then take small steps to turn. This advice holds true for outdoor work, such as raking and shoveling, too. For jobs involving lifting, from delivery work to nursing, ergonomic training is available. The Centers for Disease Control and Prevention offers a free manual on proper material handling to help reduce back, shoulder, and upper limb pain (see notes section, p. 209).

Screens — including smartphones, tablets, computers, and handheld gaming units — are all potential ergonomic nightmares. How many times have you seen a teenager hunched over their phone or a coworker slumped at their desk? *Text neck* is a real thing — pain caused by the rounded shoulders, forward-hanging head, and slouched spine associated with habitual texting. Several years ago, *Wii-itis* was a common muscle injury caused by overuse of Nintendo Wii consoles. Whatever the name, the results are the same. Poor posture, joint misalignment, asymmetrical muscle engagement, and repetitive muscle strain (from overuse or prolonged time in one position) can cause or worsen orthopaedic pain.

The solution is setting up an ergonomic work area, being mindful of your body position, and changing positions and stretching frequently. Some employers offer ergonomic evaluations of work spaces, as do physical therapists. A good ergonomic setup for computer work includes a supportive chair that adjusts so that your shoulders are relaxed, your elbows are bent, your wrists supported, your neck and spine straight and supported, your knees bent with thighs parallel to the ground, and your feet placed flat on a slightly inclined footrest. The center of your screen should be at eye level.

Even reading a book, ebook, or magazine can contribute to back, shoulder, and neck pain if it leads to poor ergonomics — hunched shoulders and a bent neck. Often, I tell my patients to use an adjustable cookbook stand, lap desk, or breakfast tray to support their reading material. Simple stretches, frequent position changes, and ergonomic awareness reduce orthopaedic pain.

CASE STUDY

Raj, a 35-year-old man, had suffered with neck pain, shoulder pain, and tingling in his arms for more than three years. The neck pain was constant, but the tingling occurred primarily at work. He spent most of the day on his computer, working as an IT specialist. He had undergone the million-dollar workup with spine and brain MRIs, blood work, and consultations with a neurologist, pain management doctor, and orthopedist. He had seen a chiropractor and tried physical therapy. These measures helped temporarily. For years, he lived on acetaminophen and topical analgesic patches that gave only minimal relief. The pain made it hard to work. He stopped golfing and even carrying his young daughter. Pain hijacked his life.

After a thorough evaluation, we determined that myofascial pain was the major cause of his pain and dysfunction. We discussed the Relief-5R plan. Raj had let self-care drop to the bottom of his to-do list as he prioritized getting ahead at work and providing for his young family. He ate fast food for lunch every day, worked long hours, and felt glued to his computer.

We identified lifestyle changes that would be easy for Raj to make. He decided to vary his lunch habits. We developed a customized two-minute stretch and exercise routine, and at work, he set a timer every hour to remind him to do it. He bought cushions for his office chair to support optimal spine alignment. He also started using an improvised standing desk that got him out of that chair regularly during the work day. Within two weeks, he felt better. He had one distinct area of muscle spasm remaining, which we treated with a trigger-point muscle injection and a new therapy program. Now, Raj does not need a timer to remind him to take stretch breaks. He habitually alternates between sitting and standing at work, takes stretch breaks when he gets up to refill his water bottle, and packs healthy leftovers for lunch. He no longer has tingling or constant neck pain. He has resumed playing golf and can carry his daughter without fear. Raj lives a life with more ease.

Movement Options

Building core strength (the muscles in the core of our body), maintaining proper joint and spine alignment, and developing solid support structures all enable us to function better with less pain. There is evidence that certain types of movement, such as yoga, water exercise, Pilates, and tai chi, reduce orthopaedic pain, and if these fit into your lifestyle, then that is great! But if not, that is okay, too. Other forms of daily and frequent movement, with a combination of aerobic and strength-building exercises, also help reduce spine, musculoskeletal, and joint pain. The goal is to increase movement in any way that works for you, from formal classes to spurts of additional activity throughout the day. Any change in your activity level should also be discussed with your physician.

Aerobic exercise is movement vigorous enough to raise our heart rate and respiratory rate for a continuous period. It improves both endurance and strength and can reduce inflammation. If you're just starting out with exercise, aim for fifteen to thirty minutes of movement at a light to moderate level, like an outdoor walk.

Strength training involves shorter bursts of repeated movements (reps) aimed at strengthening specific muscle groups. It typically involves working against resistance in the form of weights, weight machines, resistance bands, or your own body weight. It's best done every other day to allow time for your muscles to recover in between sessions. Start out with light weights or resistance, aiming to be able to do two or three sets of ten to twelve reps of each exercise (with brief rests between sets), and increase the weight as you progress.

High-intensity interval training (HIIT) involves short, intense periods of movement followed by brief recovery periods, often lasting less than fifteen minutes in total. Many people laud

HIIT as an effective and time-efficient workout. In addition, studies show that HIIT reduces inflammation and helps regulate body fat composition and blood pressure. Although many of the HIIT routines available on the internet are very challenging, there are also gentle options, including routines that can be done in a swimming pool. A study of older adults with rheumatoid arthritis found that an HIIT walking program — brief periods of rapid walking alternated with slower walking — reduced inflammation, joint swelling, and immune dysfunction. Studies involving HIIT and chronic low back pain have reported similar improvements in reducing pain and disability and increasing function.

Gravity Breaks

While daily movement helps reduce pain and inflammation, it is important to remain within your tolerance level. Many people with spine pain find gravity breaks to be extremely helpful — giving our spine and joints a break from the pressure of gravity. If possible, lie down for fifteen to twenty minutes in the middle of your day. For many retired people, a good time for a gravity break is between 2 and 3 p.m. It is a great time to practice a relaxation exercise (see chapter 6, "Refresh"), read, or watch television. If you are at work, you might have to take a mini gravity break on a mat or in your car, or lie down as soon as you get home.

The Great Outdoors

You may have noticed that I strongly recommend outdoor activities. Being outside reduces stress and inflammation and raises our mood and sense of well-being. A review study including over eight hundred young adults showed that outdoor exercise resulted in less tension, anger, and depression and a greater sense of enjoyment and well-being than indoor exercise. A mindful walk is one of the most revitalizing things you can do for yourself.

Being mindful means being present and engaging all your senses in your surroundings. In Japan, there is practice called *forest bathing*, which involves taking a mindful nature walk. You don't have to have a forest on your doorstep: the practice simply involves unplugging and reconnecting with nature. Research studies have confirmed that forest bathing reduces physical, mental, and emotional stress, lowers stress hormones, subdues the fight-or-flight system, and activates the relaxation response. All these mind-body responses help reduce chronic pain and inflammation (more on this in chapter 6, "Refresh"). Some people call outdoor exercise *green exercise*, and some physicians write prescriptions for it! No matter what we call it, outdoor activity improves our lives.

Like other living beings, humans need plenty of water, fresh air, nutrients, sunshine, rest, strong roots, and a nurturing community in order to thrive.

Revitalizing with activity improves sleep, mood, and resilience, and lowers stress. It can be an opportunity to connect with the outdoors and loved ones. The Revitalize pillar of the Relief-5R plan guides us toward a better life with less pain.

Setting Activity Goals

As with other pillars of the Relief-5R plan, microboosts can add up to big pain relief. For everyday activity, it's important to set an achievable goal. Resolving to start hiking for an hour every day may not be realistic because of time constraints, fitness level, pain, or the weather. A better goal may be committing to fifteen minutes of extra movement a day. Whatever you choose, track your activity on your phone or fitness device, or keep a journal. Make your goal specific: plan when, where, and how movement will fit into your day. Block out time for it like an appointment and, ideally, link it to a daily activity: for instance, you might resolve, "After dinner, I will walk or complete an exercise video." If you miss a day, do not give up; simply start again the next day.

After a few weeks, you will feel good about your progress and be on your way to lowering painful inflammation.

SET FOR SUCCESS: REVITALIZE

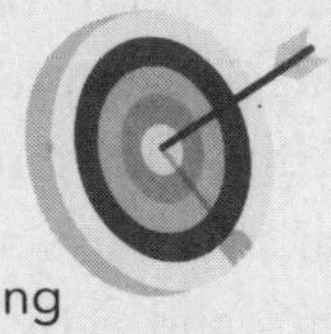

R   REMOVE BARRIERS
- **Intention:** Walk outside before driving home.
- **Microboost:** *I will put my walking shoes in the passenger seat of the car with a note that says, "Less pain."*

E   EYE LEVEL
- **Intention:** Stretch more frequently.
- **Microboost:** *I will tape a diagram of stretches next to my computer and set a timer to remind me to stretch throughout the day.*

L   LINK TO A SPECIFIC ACTIVITY
- **Intention:** Move more.
- **Microboost:** *When I drive to work or the grocery store, I will park farther away and walk.*

I   "I" DECLARATION
- **Intention:** Try an exercise video.
- **Microboost:** *Say aloud, "I will try this online video before dinner." Write on my calendar, "Try online video." I will have my phone, television, computer, or other device cued up to the video.*

E   ENCOURAGE PROGRESS BY TRACKING
- **Intention:** Keep track of my activity.
- **Microboost:** *I will dedicate a calendar or app to tracking each daily accomplishment.*

F   FEEL BETTER!

Figure 4.3. Relief-5R method for creating customized Revitalize microboosts.

Next Steps

1. Review your big goal — what you want to achieve (or prevent) by making changes.
2. From the list below, identify two microboosts that fit your life and will help you progress toward your goal.
3. Turn these microboosts into a custom Relief-5R plan with specific action steps, following the examples below.
4. Envision your big goals and know you are on your way to achieving them.
5. Feel better!

MICROBOOSTS LEVEL 1

- Use the stairs. When driving to a destination, park farther away and walk to add some extra movement to your day. If your destination is walkable, then leave the car at home.
- Block out ten or fifteen minutes for an outdoor walk.
- Make it social! Invite a friend, family member, or coworker to join you in your activity, in person or on the phone.
- Get up and walk around while talking on the phone.
- Get outside whenever you have a chance.
- Develop a list of go-to stretches or exercises for quick activity breaks.
- Set a timer to remind you to get up and move.
- While watching TV, get up and stretch during commercial breaks. If you're streaming shows without commercials, hit the pause button and take a stretch break between shows or episodes.
- Be mindful of your ergonomics at work and home, and review your computer setup for possible ergonomic improvements.
- Take a gravity break in the midafternoon or after work.

- Meet with a physical therapist to develop an activity plan that does not strain your painful area(s).
- Create a workout playlist or movie list that will encourage you to keep moving.
- Track your progress daily on a phone or log.

MICROBOOSTS LEVEL 2

- Block out time for movement on your calendar every day. Schedule a daily, twenty- to thirty-minute, moderate-intensity walk.
- Try HIIT with a free online video, app, or class.
- Consider buying or making a standing or adjustable sitting/standing desk.
- Take a class on relieving spine, musculoskeletal, or joint pain.
- Work one-on-one with a trainer.
- Add forest bathing to your routine.

CUSTOM RELIEF PLAN: EXAMPLES

- *I will walk for fifteen minutes during my lunch break.*
- *I will park farther away and walk to the grocery store and restaurants.*
- *I will get up and move during all of my phone calls.*
- *I will keep my workout clothes on top of the remote, which I will keep cued to my online workout video.*
- *I will track my progress at bedtime with stickers and a calendar.*

CHAPTER 5

Recharge

Sleep that knits up the raveled sleave of care,...
sore labor's bath,
Balm of hurt minds, great nature's second course,
Chief nourisher in life's feast.

— William Shakespeare

Myth: Sleep quality is not connected to orthopaedic pain.
Fact: Poor sleep worsens pain.
Relief-5R: Optimizing sleep is part of a pain solution.

The *rest less, work more* attitude pervades America. Skimping on sleep promises us more time, but instead it leaves us feeling unproductive and unhealthy. All-nighters, minimal sleep, and long work hours are applauded as signs of dedication among students, parents, and employees. Yet less sleep hurts us and causes more hurt. It erodes health, breeds painful inflammation, and shortens lifespan.

There are no substitutes for sleep. Skimping on sleep is akin to eating processed convenience food instead of real, nutritious food: it may feel okay in the short run, but we pay for it in the long run. Just as real food provides nutrients essential for life, sufficient sleep provides the recovery time essential to the healthy functioning of our body and brain.

Many employers — in fields ranging from law to long-distance truck driving — promote the "rest less, work more" philosophy instead of a "rest better, work better" philosophy. This leads to poorer focus, more mistakes, extra work, and damaged health. A 2020 study found that sleep deprivation can result in greater impairment than having a blood alcohol concentration over the legal driving limit. Like alcohol, too, it impairs our judgment: the same study found that drinking coffee tricked people into thinking they were more alert and less impaired than they truly were.

Sleep builds health. It allows the body to recharge and reset. It restores homeostasis (balance) and calms inflammation. Poor-quality or inadequate sleep contributes to pain, inflammation, a weakened immune system, diabetes, hypertension, heart disease, and some cancers. It feeds depression, anxiety, and other psychological disorders while decreasing focus, attention span, and memory. Poor sleep stresses the body. Recent studies suggest that insufficient sleep actually shrinks your brain: people with poor sleep quality have more cortical atrophy. Insufficient sleep decreases resilience and the ability to process and tolerate pain. Sleep deprivation leads to myriad health consequences, such as:

- increased pain
- increased inflammation
- increased stress
- increased fatigue
- decreased pain tolerance
- decreased focus
- decreased memory

- decreased brain volume
- decreased immune function
- prediabetes and diabetes
- high blood pressure
- heart disease
- mental health conditions, including depression and anxiety
- shorter healthspan
- shorter lifespan

Sleep and Inflammation

Most people know that adults typically need seven to eight hours of restorative sleep to function at their best. Shorter sleep durations (less than six hours) are correlated with higher levels of inflammation (as measured by levels of IL-6, TNF-α, and CRP). Remember how extra fat acts as an inflammation factory? Well, according to a thirteen-year study, shorter sleep duration is also associated with obesity. It is a double whammy.

The quality of our sleep matters, too. Shallow, frequently interrupted sleep is less beneficial. A 2020 study published in the *Journal of the American Medical Association* found that insufficient deep sleep is associated with a greater risk of premature death. Sufficient quality sleep is a simple, drug-free way to quell pain, reduce inflammation, and extend healthspan.

Sleep and Pain

Pain and sleep difficulties are intertwined. Pain can disrupt sleep as a result of difficulties in finding a comfortable sleeping position or experiencing pain when rolling over. Sleep can also be affected by elevated stress hormones, anxiety, and depression. In a study of people sent to pain physicians, 70 percent described their sleep as poor and reported fewer sleep hours, greater disability, higher pain levels, less daytime activity, and higher depression and anxiety scores. Poor sleep is also documented among people with rheumatoid arthritis, osteoarthritis, fibromyalgia, headaches, and other painful conditions. Even in people with and without diagnosed painful conditions, there is a clear connection between poor sleep and pain. A study of more than seventeen thousand adults found that sleeping for five hours or less per night is associated with more musculoskeletal pain.

Sleep deprivation, in turn, is known to lower pain tolerance. If you don't get enough quality sleep, you hurt more. In one study, people who slept less for ten consecutive nights were found to have higher pain levels and higher inflammatory markers. People who slept less than five hours a night not only experienced more musculoskeletal pain but also had multiple painful areas. In other words, *less sleep means more pain*. Although catching up on sleep after nights of disrupted sleep is not optimal, it still provides better pain control than NSAIDs or acetaminophen. And unlike medications and stimulants, sleep is free and free of side effects.

While night pain must always be evaluated by a physician, improving sleep is important. There is a reciprocal relationship between recharging with better sleep and the other Relief-5R pillars. SAD food choices, lack of activity, stress, and poor relationships jeopardize restorative sleep, while improving these factors improves sleep.

Conversely, if you sleep well, you are likely to make better food choices and not rely on sugar, caffeine, and processed foods to get you through the day. Recent studies show that a more diverse, healthy gut microbiome correlates with better sleep. Better sleep gives us more energy to be active, and daily movement improves sleep. Quality sleep translates to less physical and mental stress as well as more resilience for coping with pain and difficult situations. In turn, reducing stress and focusing on positive relationships improves your sense of well-being and your sleep. All the relief factors interconnect.

Sleep and Hormones

Hormones are regulatory, signaling substances that help maintain homeostasis (balance) in the body. While many hormones affect sleep, we will focus on the five listed below.

- **Cortisol**, our old friend, the stress hormone, helps us wake up and be alert in the morning.
- **Melatonin** relaxes us in preparation for sleep.
- **Leptin** decreases appetite (makes us feel full).
- **Ghrelin** increases appetite (makes us feel hungry).
- **Growth hormone** aids in tissue repair and growth during sleep.

Our circadian rhythm rules the natural sleep-wake cycle. We want to program our internal clocks to maximize quality sleep and healing time. Exposure to natural light in the morning is best, if possible. Bright light not only triggers the release of cortisol but also triggers a melatonin surge fourteen to sixteen hours later. This coincides with the fading of natural daylight. In the evening, it is better to follow this pattern and use dimmer light and desk lamps as opposed to bright, overhead lighting. Unfortunately, screen use before bedtime disrupts the release of melatonin, leading to poorer sleep and recovery. As melatonin levels increases, our cortisol levels should decrease. However, lingering stress from the day or stressful entertainment, news or conversations close to bedtime can elevate cortisol levels. A relaxation routine helps us ride the melatonin wave and unwind in preparation for sleep.

Insufficient sleep creates a hormonal downward spiral by raising cortisol levels, thereby increasing inflammation, pain, dis-ease, and other stress responses. In addition, cortisol lowers our levels of leptin, the hormone that helps regulate appetite by making us feel full, and increases levels of ghrelin, the hunger hormone. This disruption of the hormones that influence when and how much we eat may explain the documented correlation between poor sleep and higher body weight. This all leads to more eating, more fatty inflammatory tissue, and more painful inflammation.

Growth hormone, primarily produced at night, plays an important role in food processing, maintenance of muscle mass, and bone health, as well as tissue repair and growth. Poor sleep disrupts growth hormone production. This translates to less healing, decreased muscle mass, and poorer bone health. All of these factors contribute to more pain and inflammation.

It makes sense. If we skimp on one kind of fuel (sleep), we attempt to compensate with another kind of fuel (food). But the two are not interchangeable. More food (even healthy food) is an inadequate remedy for insufficient sleep. Instead of providing the body with an opportunity to rest and recharge, we inundate it with more work in the forms of information processing and food metabolizing. Our body may be pleading, in the famous words of Nell Carter, "Gimme a break."

Strategic Napping

Many of us try to catch up on sleep lost during the week by sleeping late on weekends and vacation days. But sleeping in does not recoup all the benefits of lost sleep. One study looking at people who slept less during the week and extra on the weekends showed that these people ate more food after dinner, increased their body weight, disrupted their circadian rhythm, and reduced their body's insulin sensitivity. The consequences of less weekday sleep are eating more food, gaining weight, increasing blood sugar, increasing inflammation, and disrupting your body's natural rhythm. A schedule that allows for seven to nine hours of high-quality sleep is more beneficial than late rising on weekends.

Life happens, of course, and sleep may suffer. When that happens, to nap or to not nap? That is the question. The answer is: it depends. If you miss an hour or more of your night's sleep, your mood and mental function may benefit from a nap, but keep a few guidelines in mind. Your goal is still to sleep for seven to nine hours in a twenty-four-hour period. Data suggest that excessive sleep can be detrimental, too. In addition, naps may disrupt your nighttime sleep.

Nap if you need to, but avoid napping late in the day (after 3 p.m.), and aim to nap for no more than twenty to thirty minutes. Skip the nap if you have trouble sleeping at night.

Unwinding: A Bedtime Relaxation Routine

If sleep is so important, does it make sense to take sleeping pills? Unfortunately, sleep medications often result in poorer sleep. They carry a risk of dependency, addiction, harmful side effects, and interactions with other medications or substances.

An excellent nonmedication sleep aid is cognitive behavior therapy for insomnia (CBT-I). Like other forms of cognitive CBT, it involves consciously identifying and changing negative thoughts and behavior. CBT-I has been found to lengthen sleep time, improve sleep quality, and reduce pain; it has even been recommended as a way to decrease postoperative opioid use. However, this approach takes time and commitment.

Let's consider a do-it-yourself CBT-I approach: establishing a bedtime relaxation routine. We thrive on routines, and our bodies respond to cues synced with our circadian rhythm. Many parents sleep-train their children by establishing a regular bedtime routine that may include a bath, brushing teeth, and story time. Adults can benefit from a similar approach.

Common ways to improve sleep without medication focus on sleep hygiene, stimulus control, and limiting daytime napping. Sleep hygiene means improving our sleep habits by changing our attitudes toward sleep, practicing sleep-inducing behaviors, tracking our sleep, and avoiding stimulation before bedtime. Stimulus control means treating our bed as a place associated only with sleep (and intimacy), not with eating, working, or watching television. Below we will examine several components of a bedtime relaxation routine that enhances sleep and helps us wake up refreshed and ready to face the day.

Circadian Eating

Eating and sleeping in sync with our circadian rhythms enhances our well-being. Circadian eating also provides a buffer between digestion and sleep time. Avoiding food close to bedtime reduces stress on the body and digestive problems such as reflux, and it gives the body more time and resources for repair. Studies have found that eating near bedtime results in higher calorie consumption and more potential weight gain, which can increase painful inflammation.

Other things to avoid for several hours before bedtime are tobacco, alcohol, caffeinated beverages, and other stimulants. Because the stimulant effects of caffeine are persistent, most people benefit from avoiding caffeine after noon. Alcohol also disrupts quality sleep. Although it may make some people feel sleepy or fall asleep, it does not deliver pain-fighting, restorative sleep. It is best to limit or avoid alcohol.

Limiting other fluid intake within two hours of bedtime can also minimize sleep disruption by reducing bathroom visits — but this is beneficial only if you are well hydrated, have no other medical conditions, and have been drinking water throughout the day.

Creating a Low-Stress Zone

Your bedroom should make you feel calm, cool, and relaxed, not alert and wired. It should be a sanctuary that induces a sense of serenity and well-being, a place that cues your brain for sleep. This means, as much as possible, keeping work out of your bedroom. Even if you live in a studio apartment or shared room, avoid using your phone or laptop in bed.

To prepare for sleep, it is also important to avoid stimulating TV shows, stressful news, and tough conversations (in person or on the phone) at bedtime. Stress pumps up the fight-or-flight system and leaves you wired long after the discussion has ended. Try to make the last ninety minutes of your day drama-free time. This may not always be possible with children, spouses, roommates, and work commitments, but even if another person pushes your buttons, you can temper your response in order to support your bedtime relaxation routine.

Keep your bedroom cool, quiet, and dark — a sleep cave. While temperature preferences vary, try to keep your bedroom cool enough to make snuggling under a sheet or blanket inviting. If you share a bed, having your own cover sheet and blanket or duvet can avoid a nightly tug-of-war. A fan can circulate cool air and provide some consistent white noise. If you can't control the noise level, consider white noise or ear plugs. Similarly, keeping the room dark promotes better sleep. If you live in a place with short summer nights or work a night shift, try blackout curtains or an eye mask. Make your sleep cave a relaxing, inviting sleep spot that helps you recover, recharge, and reduce pain.

Creating a Low-Electronic Zone (and Avoiding "Revenge Bedtime Procrastination")

It's not just the stimulating or stressful content brought to us by electronic devices that can interfere with bedtime relaxation; the blue light emitted by their screens has been shown to disrupt melatonin release. In an ideal world, we would ban electronics for ninety minutes before bedtime. All right, we live in the real world. We can start by avoiding phones, screens, and other electronic devices for thirty minutes before bedtime. Many sleep experts recommend leaving your smartphone outside your bedroom. If you can do this and charge your phone overnight in another room, that is fantastic! But many of us need to keep our phone handy in case of emergencies, and we also use it as our alarm clock. The second problem is easy to solve. An old-fashioned, inexpensive alarm clock will prevent middle-of-the-night time checks on a bright, stimulating phone screen and save you from pondering (if not opening) an email or other notification. If the light from a digital clock disturbs your sleep or the numbers hypnotize you, face the clock away from you. It will be there when you need it and is infinitely better than checking the time on your phone at night. Some digital clocks also offer soothing sounds to help you fall asleep.

If you cannot leave your phone in another room, it helps to put the phone on silent mode or airplane mode or even turn it off. If you use the phone to listen to a bedtime relaxation recording or white noise, place it at arm's length or face down to remove it from immediate view.

If you cannot avoid screen use within ninety minutes of bedtime, consider wearing inexpensive amber-tinted glasses. These lenses block the blue light from screens so that melatonin can work its magic. In studies, people who wore amber lenses two hours before bedtime for only one week reported increases in sleep time, quality, and soundness. It is still important to try to designate the last thirty minutes before bedtime as screen-free time.

Another reason to avoid bedtime screen use is that it sets the stage for "revenge bedtime procrastination." This nasty but widespread habit means staying up later and sacrificing sleep to do something leisurely that we feel cheated out of doing during the day. Often, this involves binge-watching shows, shopping, or scrolling through endless social media feeds. It provides a release of feel-good chemicals in our brains and feels like a well-deserved treat after a long day of working, taking care of others, and simply surviving. Unfortunately, this "treat" dooms us to more stress, pain, and inflammation. To help remove this temptation, avoid screen use before bedtime and replace it with a nightly practice that truly nourishes you, leading to more rest and less stress.

Practicing Gratitude

Once you've put down your phone, laptop, or remote control, bedtime is a great time for a gratitude practice. Positive bedtime thoughts help conquer worries and negative thinking. Focusing on the good things in your life sets you up for higher-quality sleep. Many people advocate writing down three things you are thankful for each day. These don't have to be exceptional: they might include the smell of fresh flowers at the grocery store, your friend's goofy, snort-filled laugh, or the calmness of an evening walk. If this sounds like too much, start by identifying one thing each day. Think of just one moment in your day when you felt good, and write it down.

Being grateful at bedtime has been shown to improve sleep quality and duration, and reduce the time it takes to fall asleep. In the Refresh and Relate chapters, we will dig deeper into the pain-relieving effects of gratitude and discover more gratitude microboosts. For now, I recommend Irving Berlin's sage advice: "If you... can't sleep, just count your blessings instead of sheep."

Mindfulness and Meditation

In addition to a gratitude practice during your thirty-minute, screen-free time before bed, you can try a relaxation method to calm your mind. Bedtime mindfulness and meditation practices have been shown to improve the quality of sleep and decrease depression, insomnia, and anxiety. They also give you a head start on the next day by improving mood, boosting energy, and building pain resilience.

A relaxation routine might include meditation, mindfulness, soothing prayers, breathing techniques, muscle relaxation exercises, or writing in a journal. Use any method that helps you let go of the day's stresses.

Many free or inexpensive meditation, mindfulness, and relaxation apps and recordings are available and may be helpful.

Using these is one exception to the rule about avoiding device use before bedtime, but if you use an app on your phone, try putting the phone in airplane mode to avoid distractions, and turn the screen off or place the phone face down.

A simple meditation that requires no electronic device entails slow, relaxed breathing, making your exhalation longer than your inhalation, while repeating a simple version of the traditional loving-kindness meditation: *May I have ease. May I have calm. May I have peace.* (There's more on this in chapter 6, "Refresh".) Give it try now: repeat it to yourself three times with your eyes closed or lowered and see how it feels.

Some people find that troubling thoughts pop up at bedtime. If your mind keeps racing with worries, to-do lists, or fears, off-load these thoughts from your brain by putting them on paper. After writing everything down, read the to-dos and prioritize them. Then try to reframe them. If you are worried that you have too much to do the next day, remind yourself that you have a checklist, you know what you want to do first, and you will do everything better if you sleep well. If you are having serious trouble managing these worries, consider talking to your physician and a therapist.

Getting Ready to Roll

For a better day with less pain and more energy, preparation starts the night before. Waking up ready to roll is easier if we prepare for the next morning's chores before bedtime. Knowing that things are in order for the next day clears our minds for restful sleep. Planning our wardrobe and our morning routine reduces "morning decision fatigue" and the stress of rushing to get everyone in the household ready for work or school on time. Decide what you want to drink in the morning — coffee or tea? — and set the timer on your coffee maker so that your coffee is ready when you reach the kitchen, or place the tea bag next to your mug on the counter, ready to go. Pick out your clothes for the next day. Set out breakfast items. If you pack a lunch, prepare and refrigerate it the night before. Build a little extra time into your routine to allow at least five minutes of mindfulness or meditation practice — and time to cope with mishaps. A morning plan is a path to freedom from stress, inflammation, and pain.

Another way to start your day off right and with less pain is to avoid looking at your phone for the first thirty minutes you are awake. The morning sets the tone for your whole day, and self-care should be your number one priority — not your employer's emails, random social media posts, or a news broadcast. The first ten minutes of my day are dedicated to prayer, gratitude, and a loving-kindness meditation. Gratitude and calmness bookend my day to start me out in a good, low-stress place and help me return to it at night. This lowers stress, inflammation, and pain. The 30/30 plan of no screens thirty minutes before bedtime and thirty minutes after rising guides us to more relief.

Sleep Tracking

Sleep does not happen in isolation from your daily activities. Tracking your sleep, along with other habits and practices, can help you develop an effective sleep plan. Some wearable fitness devices can monitor your sleep, but it's possible to do it without technology, too. Tracking your sleep, including the time you lay down, whether you had trouble falling or staying asleep, and when you woke up the next day, will help you uncover patterns and identify factors that affect your sleep. For example, many people sleep better on days when they complete thirty minutes of movement. You may also notice the negative impact of extra caffeine, alcohol, or a stressful bedtime discussion. Review this tracking data regularly and use it to refine your relaxation routine.

Pulling It Together

Other integrative methods to promote sleep may be added to your relaxation routine as well. Natural approaches are best. Some people benefit from melatonin or magnesium supplements, but levels of both can be increased simply by incorporating more real foods into your diet, especially at dinnertime. Other possibly beneficial diet additions and supplements include chamomile tea, ashwagandha, vitamin B12, and tryptophan. Before considering a supplement or advanced treatment, discuss it with your physician. Below is a list of common integrative sleep methods to explore further if needed:

- mindfulness
- meditation
- breathing techniques
- yoga
- progressive muscle relaxation
- body scan
- acupuncture
- CBT-I
- guided imagery
- massage
- lavender aromatherapy
- melatonin (nuts, fruits, vegetables, olive oil)
- magnesium (legumes, nuts, seeds, spinach)
- vitamin B12
- tryptophan
- taurine
- chamomile tea
- ashwagandha

The RELIEF tool can help you customize the microboosts that work best for you and your schedule.

SET FOR SUCCESS: RECHARGE

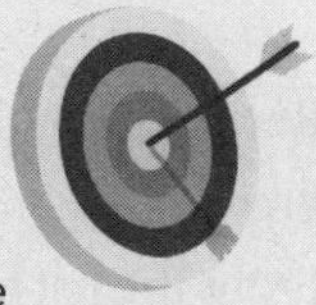

R   REMOVE BARRIERS
- **Intention:** Try a mindfulness exercise at bedtime.
- **Microboost:** *I will place a mindfulness book on my nightstand.*

E   EYE LEVEL
- **Intention:** Make a list of things that I am grateful for each night.
- **Microboost:** *I will keep an inviting notebook or gratitude journal next to my bed with a pen.*

L   LINK TO A SPECIFIC ACTIVITY
- **Intention:** Avoid screens at bedtime for better sleep.
- **Microboost:** *After I brush my teeth, I will put my phone out of reach on the dresser.*

I   "I" DECLARATION
- **Intention:** Make my bedroom a relaxing sleep sanctuary.
- **Microboost:** *Say aloud, "I will not have stressful conversations in my bedroom." Write down, "I will not work in my bedroom." Place my favorite relaxation tools (book, scented oil, massage roller, or relaxing music player) next to the bed.*

E   ENCOURAGE PROGRESS BY TRACKING
- **Intention:** Keep track of my sleep habits to improve sleep quality.
- **Microboost:** *I will dedicate a calendar or app to tracking caffeine intake, bedtime relaxation routine, and sleep quality.*

F.   FEEL BETTER!

Figure 5.1. Relief-5R method for creating customized Recharge microboosts.

Next Steps

1. Review your big goal — what you want to achieve (or prevent) by making changes.
2. From the list below, identify two microboosts that fit your life and will help you progress toward your goal.
3. Turn these microboosts into a custom Relief-5R plan with specific action steps, following the examples below.
4. Envision your big goals and know you are on your way to achieving them.
5. Feel better!

MICROBOOSTS LEVEL 1

- Prioritize sleep by scheduling eight to nine hours in bed.
- Stick to a consistent sleep schedule.
- Build a cozy sleep cave: a low-electronic and low-stress zone.
- Consider buying a low-blue-light alarm clock instead of using your phone.
- Get some bright outdoor light in the morning to set your circadian timer.
- Increase daily movement for better sleep (see the list of Revitalize microboosts in chapter 4, p. 100).
- Limit naps to twenty to thirty minutes while keeping in mind the goal of seven to nine hours of total sleep over a twenty-four-hour period.
- Restrict caffeine intake after noon.
- Eat a variety of colorful vegetables and fruits for a balanced gut microbiome and better sleep.
- Avoid tobacco, alcohol, and stimulants within three to six hours of bedtime.
- Limit what goes into your mouth close to bedtime.

- Avoid screens for *at least* thirty minutes before bedtime.
- Adopt the 30/30 plan: no screens thirty minutes before bedtime and for the first thirty minutes in the morning.
- Pick a relaxation technique to practice during the screen-free time.
- Offload and write down bedtime worries, to-do items, and thoughts.
- Reserve time for evening gratitude.
- Try a no-tech bedtime mantra: *May I have ease. May I have calm. May I have peace.*

Microboosts Level 2

- Try tracking your sleep, activities, fuel, and stressors throughout the day to identify actions and events that trigger poor sleep.
- If you must look at screens within ninety minutes of bedtime, consider wearing amber lenses.
- Set yourself up to be ready to roll the next morning.
- Avoid bright overhead light after sunset; stick to dimmer desk or table lamps.
- Discuss integrative methods for improving sleep with your healthcare provider.
- Consider consultation with a trained CBT-I specialist.

Custom Relief Plan: Examples

- *I will not have caffeine after noon at home or work.*
- *I will avoid screens for thirty minutes before bed.*
- *I will practice my favorite relaxation technique or read before bedtime.*
- *I will think of one person, one place, and one thing that I am grateful for while I brush my teeth.*

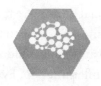

CHAPTER 6

Refresh

*During my own years of chronic pain, I suffered much more from my
thoughts — "I can't bear this!" "It will last forever!" "I'll never have
a normal life!" — than from the actual physical sensations....Your
thoughts, even thoughts you absolutely believe, may not always be true.*

— Martha Beck

Myth: Stress and pain expectations do not affect
　　orthopaedic pain.

Fact: Stress and a poor mindset worsen orthopaedic
　　pain and inflammation.

Relief-5R: Lowering stress and ending suffering is part
　　of a true pain solution.

Our pain level and suffering depend on more than physical
health. The people around us and our environment all affect
our pain experience. A true pain solution takes a biopsychoso-
cial approach to pain, one that recognizes the whole person and
addresses psychological and social as well as biological factors.

Unfortunately, conventional healthcare tends to focus on physical stressors (such as injury and disease agents) and treats mental and emotional stress like unwanted stepchildren. Yet all three types of stress can spike painful inflammation. Every medical condition I have encountered may be caused or worsened by emotional and mental stress, from muscle spasms and disc pain to heartburn and diabetes.

In fact, mental and emotional stress not only aggravate chronic pain but also create suffering. *Pain* is usually defined as the unpleasant physical sensations of an injury or condition, while *suffering* is a combination of the physical symptoms, emotional burden, and mental burden. Often, suffering translates to a negative distortion in a person's self-image and planned life narrative. Even without a definitive physical injury, mental and emotional stress can manifest as pain, spasms, and suffering. For many of us, simply thinking about a stressful event, an unsupportive boss, or a particular politician tightens our muscles. Our shoulders tense, our heart pumps faster, and our breathing quickens. Pain and inflammation start to rise.

We all have pain at times, but we do not have to suffer. When stress hits us, we can use techniques such as breathing exercises and visualizations of somebody we love to release some of the tension and slow the painful inflammation train. There are also many steps we can take to lower our ongoing stress and build resilience. We can live better by tackling physical, mental, and emotional stress with Refresh microboosts.

Pain, Inflammation, and the Brain

Stress triggers the fight-or-flight response. It saves our lives in dangerous situations like facing a fire or robber because it prompts us to act immediately, without pausing to think. But modern life activates this same quick reaction to nonthreatening and threatening situations — from dealing with a screaming toddler, a reckless driver, or a frustrated customer to handling an irate boss, a nagging partner, or a devastating medical condition. Under repetitive and ongoing stress, we default to immediate, emotional reactions. Many of us are living our lives on a hair trigger, ready to fight, flight or freeze in response to the slightest challenge (figure 6.1).

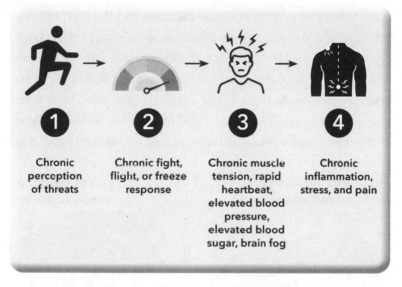

1	2	3	4
Chronic perception of threats	Chronic fight, flight, or freeze response	Chronic muscle tension, rapid heartbeat, elevated blood pressure, elevated blood sugar, brain fog	Chronic inflammation, stress, and pain

Figure 6.1. Chronic stress response.

With this chronic activation, our muscles tense and our blood sugar spikes. Our immune system, which is meant to protect us, treats our body as the enemy. Our entire body shifts to a state of ongoing panic, pain, and inflammation.

Chronic stress reconfigures our brain, weakening our higher-level brain functions — thought, attention, and behavior. This is the "thrive" part of the brain, which enables us to handle challenges and build pain resilience. Stress impairs this evolved part of the brain and expands connections to the emotional, primitive part of the brain. As a result, the emotional response wins out in challenging situations. That's why we snap at a child's hundredth question, swear at the person who cuts us off in traffic, or get defensive with an annoying coworker. Often stress-induced anger, fear, or desperation leads us to say something we did not mean, or at least would not have said aloud if we were calmer. Daily, repeated stress reinforces this response and makes it a reflex. If we hear our child start to whine, our heart rate increases. If somebody cuts ahead of us in traffic, our jaw clenches, and the survival brain activates. If a customer starts yelling at us, we start yelling back. Our goal is to be able to handle a challenge with a rational *response* and not a knee-jerk *reaction*. Over time, connections to the thrive brain dwindle while those to the survival brain grow. With these changes, our pain tolerance and hope for recovery diminish. Every little stressor causes pain, and recovery feels impossible (figure 6.2).

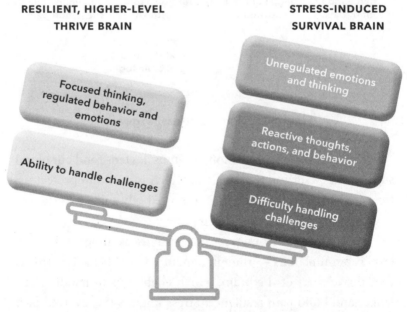

RESILIENT, HIGHER-LEVEL THRIVE BRAIN

STRESS-INDUCED SURVIVAL BRAIN

Focused thinking, regulated behavior and emotions

Ability to handle challenges

Unregulated emotions and thinking

Reactive thoughts, actions, and behavior

Difficulty handling challenges

Figure 6.2. Chronic stress leads to domination by the survival brain.

Most people recognize the connection between stress and pain. In one study, Americans reported that the number one cause of their low back pain was stress. When we are stressed, our muscles tighten and our pain tolerance plummets. In addition, chronic stress (mental, social, or physical) can manifest as physical pain. Most orthopaedic pain has a myofascial component (based in muscle tissue). It can be due to local injury or protective spasm; it can also result from stress. Pain caused or aggravated by chronic stress is self-reinforcing, because chronic fight-or-flight activation shunts blood to larger organs and away from smaller muscles, supporting tissues, and nerves. This results in less oxygen and nutrient flow to many of our painful areas.

Studies have proved that psychosocial stress (including interpersonal conflict, being a caregiver, martial problems, social isolation, perceived stress, and depression) results in weight gain and elevated markers of inflammation, including IL-6 and CRP. Similarly, needy and difficult relationships stress the body and manifest themselves as inflammation and pain. In a 2020 study, when healthy people were placed under acute psychosocial stress, they were found to have a lower tolerance for pain. Both acute and ongoing stressors can reduce pain tolerance. To make matters worse, stress not only aggravates pain but also makes it harder to handle painful situations.

Despite these findings, typical pain treatments still rely on anti-inflammatory medications. These temporarily block the body's pain signals but do not tackle any of the causes of the pain. If we are living in survival mode, we cannot heal, repair, or recover from pain. The Refresh pain solution improves our stress response by altering our pain mindset. While we may not be able to avoid stressful situations or people, we can improve the ways we approach and process these challenges.

The Relief-5R Connection

All of the pillars of the Relief-5R plan interconnect and reinforce each other, for better or worse. Insufficient sleep increases our cortisol levels and fuels more stress, anxiety, and despair. Stress leads to poor food choices, difficulty sleeping, and more pain. Cortisol also lowers our levels of leptin (the feeling-full hormone) and often leads to eating more. As noted, a longitudinal study confirmed an association between additional weight gain and psychological stress related to work demands, financial strain, family relationships, depression, and anxiety. During stressful times, we often not only eat more food overall but eat more sugar-laden, fatty, and processed foods. These are known as "comfort" foods for a reason: they temporarily dupe our bodies into feeling better. In the long run, however, they cause more inflammation and pain — which can in turn lead us to try to comfort ourselves with more unhealthy foods. In this cruel cycle, stress leads to poor food choices, more weight gain, poorer nutrition, and more painful inflammation.

Chronic stress also changes our gut microbiome, and this affects our inflammation, pain, and mood. We have to free ourselves from this harmful pain cycle by reducing stress and building resilience. With our hectic lives, we may feel we lack time, energy, or money to dedicate to stress relief. But there is an easy way to break the cycle of stress, inflammation, and pain with a small commitment of time and no monetary cost.

Deeper Dive: Telomeres

Stress reduces our lifespan in multiple ways. One of these is the damage it does to our telomeres, the caps on the ends of our chromosomes that protect our DNA from damage. Telomeres shorten with aging and oxidative stress, making our cells less able to repair themselves and regenerate. Stress, smoking, obesity, lack of movement, and an unhealthy diet accelerate telomere damage, increasing the risk of death from heart disease, some degenerative diseases, and cancer. But this process can be slowed and to some degree reversed. The Relief-5R plan helps preserve and protect telomeres. Refresh microboosts like mindfulness meditation may increase telomere length and can decrease painful inflammation.

Healing Mind and Body

No matter how much conventional healthcare tries to chop us up into organ systems, we are one interconnected person. In particular, it is ludicrous to treat the mind and body as separate. Stressors affect the mind and body simultaneously, and our mental and physical states affect each other. Thankfully, this holds true for stress-relieving activities as well as harmful ones. An activity or practice that boosts well-being benefits the whole person, mind and body. Going for a hike not only improves musculoskeletal and cardiac health but also supports a healthy and resilient mind.

We can take advantage of this connection and reduce physical pain with practices designed to tackle mental and emotional stress. Calming our mind helps relieve stress and pain in our body. So how do we take advantage of the mind-body connection?

The natural antidote to the stress response is the relaxation response, part of the parasympathetic nervous system, that stops the release of stress hormones and replaces them with hormones that relax us and enhance our sense of well-being. Our heart rate and breathing slow down, our blood pressure drops, and our tense muscles relax. By intentionally triggering our relaxation response several times every day, we can calm our body down from a constant, stressful state of high alert.

EFFECTS OF THE RELAXATION RESPONSE
- lowers heart rate
- lowers blood pressure

- slows breathing
- relaxes tight, painful muscles
- increases blood flow to painful areas
- decreases painful inflammation
- improves pain coping skills
- supports clear, rational thinking
- reduces emotional outbursts

Below we'll take a look at some ways to activate the relaxation response.

Adult Time-Outs

Mind-body activities such as mindfulness, meditation, yoga, breathing exercises, tai chi, and qigong have been conclusively shown to decrease pain, stress, and inflammation at the molecular level. But activating the relaxation response does not require a commitment to a formal practice. The easy way to do it is by spending at least ten minutes a day doing something joyful that engages both your body and your mind — meditating, doodling, walking outside, taking a warm bath, reading a magazine, or enjoying any other screen-free activity. Although these activities may appear to have no practical purpose or goal, they have a vital, powerful role in relieving stress and pain and building resilience. Got ten minutes?

Remember as kids, how we dreaded nap times, early bedtimes, and time-outs? Now, as adults, we crave these breaks. A ten-minute break to destress is just what the doctor ordered. Let's call it an adult time-out (ATO). During an ATO, you don't have to answer to anybody, perform, produce, or achieve. Don't worry about what has to be done or what didn't get done; simply be present with the experience and your senses. As with any new skill, relaxation grows easier with practice.

The following list offers some suggestions for ATO activities. Below we look at some of these in more detail.

ADULT TIME-OUT ACTIVITIES

- mindfulness in daily activity (walking, eating, listening)
- meditation, including guided imagery and progressive muscle relaxation
- breathing exercises
- gratitude practice
- self-massage and acupressure
- yoga, tai chi, qigong
- listening to music
- reading
- walking in nature
- dancing
- drawing, painting, coloring, doodling
- journaling
- writing a letter, thank-you note, or email
- cooking
- calling a friend
- connecting with a neighbor
- playing with a pet

Meditation and Mindfulness

Even if chronic stress has taken its toll, there are techniques we can use to repair the damage. Mindfulness and meditation practices decrease inflammation, boost immunity, and protect telomeres. These techniques can reduce the need for opioids and other pain medications.

Mindfulness is the practice of being present, aware, and engaged in whatever you are doing. It is about accepting the present — good, bad, and ugly — rather than dwelling on the past or future. Meditation is a way of practicing mindfulness that usually involves focusing inward on the breath, a mantra, or an image to decrease mental chatter and the tendency to pass judgment. The unifying theme of these practices is being present in the current moment and reducing distracting, racing thoughts.

A review of more than thirty studies found that after only a few weeks, meditation decreased levels of the inflammatory markers CRP and IL-6. A study of US marines found decreased stress markers in the group that received mindfulness training versus the group that did not receive this training. Multiple studies have demonstrated that mindfulness and meditation techniques decrease low back pain, chronic pain, and fibromyalgia pain. In fact, mindfulness and meditation can help relieve all the chronic conditions listed below — for free, with no side effects!

CHRONIC CONDITIONS RELIEVED BY MEDITATION AND MINDFULNESS

- chronic pain
- low back pain
- muscle tension
- fibromyalgia
- headaches
- depression
- anxiety
- cognitive dysfunction
- heart disease
- obesity
- high cholesterol
- psoriasis

These practices also restore and refresh the mind. Studies have shown that after a dedicated eight-week mindfulness program, the part of the brain involved in learning, memory, perspective, and emotional control actually grows! And the benefits are long-lasting. A study of adults with chronic low back pain who took part in an eight-week mindfulness program found not only that their pain decreased during the program but that the benefits continued for a year after the course.

Even better, these practices show benefits even without large time commitments. Once we learn the practice, we can lower stress and painful inflammation by investing ten to fifteen minutes in ourselves daily.

Benefits of Meditation and Mindfulness

- less pain
- less muscle tightness
- less inflammation
- lower blood sugar
- lower blood pressure
- less stress
- less anxiety
- less depression
- better sleep
- better immune function
- better telomere health
- better focus and attention
- better mood
- better quality of life
- longer lifespan
- longer healthspan

Mindfulness and meditation cultivate awareness of your current physical, emotional, and mental states. In difficult situations, this awareness can help you pause and respond in a considered way.

Spotlight: Mindfulness

Mindfulness enables us to be present and assess our internal and external situation. This allows us to respond to a stressor instead of just reacting to it. It helps develop a calmness that is not easily disrupted by outside factors. For example, if you have been waiting on hold on the phone for several minutes, you may start to feel angry. You may even think, "I am angry." After another two minutes, you switch into Hulk mode. The stress reaction switches on, your survival brain takes over, and you are ready to fight. Charged with emotion, you may yell at and alienate the person who takes your call instead of eliciting their cooperation.

We do not have to be possessed by our emotions. Mindfulness and meditation help us recognize the feeling of anger, and pause before it triggers a full-on fight-or-flight reaction. This pause lets us respond more calmly, preventing the release of stress hormones that can fuel painful inflammation.

A mindfulness practice involves being present and engaging your senses. Small children have an intuitive knowledge of how to be in the moment — not concerned with the future or past. For example, a child playing in a sandbox is completely engaged in what she is doing. She feels the sand tickle her toes. She smiles at the sound of wet sand plopping into a bucket. She does not fret about homework, chores, or a toy she lost yesterday. She is immersed in the present experience. As adults, we may have similar experiences when we engage in a favorite activity, like playing an instrument, exercising, or cooking. It is often called being in a "flow state" or "being in the zone."

Mindfulness includes microboosts such as a relaxation practice, screen-free ATOs, and avoiding multitasking. Screens are a constant source of input and a distraction from being present. More screen time correlates with obesity and more inflammation. Mealtime screen time robs us of interaction, enjoyment of our food, and engagement in the moment. It puts our brain on autopilot as we mindlessly shovel food into our mouths. A simple remedy is to make dinnertime screen-free: no phones, devices, or television. A way to double down on this positive change is to start dinner with a conversation about something good that happened that day. If you are dining solo, it could be a time to reflect on a positive event in your day or a moment of gratitude.

Eating while staring at a screen is a form of multitasking — trying to accomplish multiple tasks at once in the name of efficiency. The concept originates from computer terminology. But whereas computers can efficiently process multiple operations at once, our brains cannot. We can do several things at the same time (or, more accurately, in rapid alternation), but we cannot do them well. We are less productive when we multitask and often do not even realize it. Switching between two tasks is called *mental juggling*. It uses more energy than focusing on one task at a time, takes longer, and impairs performance. If you are listening to music and chopping vegetables, you will probably survive with all your fingers intact. But if one or both tasks require higher-level thinking, or if a small error leads to a dangerous consequence, then mental juggling spells trouble. The clearest example of this is cell phone use and driving. There is abundant data showing that mentally juggling between these tasks can lead to deadly consequences.

In addition to impairing our performance of tasks, multitasking can be bad for our physical and mental health. Responding to multiple stimuli at the same time is stressful and results in increased heart rate, blood pressure, and perceived workload. Multitasking stresses our bodies, makes us feel like we have more work, and contributes to burnout, anxiety, and depression. This increases painful inflammation.

When you have a choice, avoid multitasking. It may mean getting up a little bit earlier in the day to get some things done, asking for help, saying no to requests, or cutting yourself some slack, but the payoff is less stress and less painful inflammation. Having a schedule with enough time built in for completing specific tasks, transitions, relaxation, and human connection reduces stress and gives us the grace and time to be human.

A simple way to begin practicing mindfulness is to apply it to a common daily activity — such as walking, eating, listening to someone speak, or completing chores — paying attention to the sounds and sensations of the activity as you experience them. Examples are shown in figure 6.3. Sometimes the mind wanders during a mindfulness activity. If it does, gently but firmly guide it back to the present moment.

Being present without having to go anywhere, answer to anybody, or be "on" builds our mental and emotional reserves. It allows us to handle pain better and eliminate suffering.

Mindfulness in Daily Activities

WALKING

- What sounds do you hear? (Birds singing, cars, people)
- What do you smell? (Fresh flowers, pine sap, street vendor food)
- What does your skin feel? (Cool breeze, crisp air, warm wind)
- What do you see? (Squirrels running, ants climbing, billboards flashing)

EATING

- What does the food feel like against your teeth and tongue?
- What does it sound like?
- What do you smell?
- What flavors do you taste?
- What colors do you see on your plate?

LISTENING

- What does the speaker sound like?
- What are they telling you with their expressions and body language?
- Can you listen without trying to think of a response?
- Can you silently use eye contact, nod, or smile to show that you are engaged?
- Can you wait to speak until they pause or ask for a response?

SITTING

- Sit in a comfortable position with your feet on the ground.
- Close your eyes or lower your gaze to the ground.
- Can you feel the chair and ground supporting you?
- How does the air feel entering through your nose and leaving through your mouth?
- How does your body feel?

Figure 6.3. Adding mindfulness to daily activities.

CASE STUDY

Anita, a 52-year-old woman, had suffered with spasms and tightness in her neck and shoulders for more than a year. The constant tightness, punctuated by episodes when her neck locked up, drained her. Pain limited even her ability to drive, making it difficult to back out of a parking space or check for cars before changing lanes. For months, she sought relief with ibuprofen and heating pads, with little improvement. Anita worked from home in endless pain. She stopped playing tennis and driving on busy roads, and she worried that she might have a flare at any moment. She felt on edge all the time and snapped at her family daily. She stopped living her life fully.

Anita had tried physical therapy once but quit because she feared it might aggravate her pain. After seeing several specialists and having multiple MRIs, she was told her only options were medications: muscle relaxers and painkillers. By the time she came to see me, she felt doomed. Painful suffering had robbed her of joy, exercise, freedom, and peaceful family time.

Anita recognized that stress made her pain worse, so we discussed the Relief-5R plan and reviewed some of her stressors, such as interacting with her teenage children and trying to impress her new boss. We talked about the connection between stress and painful inflammation. Anita decided to try a mindfulness program. In fact, her employer offered employees a free mindfulness phone application. She committed to practicing mindfulness with this app for ten minutes a day for four weeks. The first week, Anita did not notice any difference, but she stuck with it. After two weeks, she found herself looking forward to this downtime and practiced in the morning before her kids were awake. This adult time-out started her day on a refreshing note, and she felt better prepared to handle work and other demands. After four weeks, she reported that she had had no major flare-ups and did not need daily ibuprofen. We added some stretches and topical treatments to her morning routine, along with some other microboosts, and at her next visit she still had experienced no flares. Her neck and shoulder tightness had decreased, and on most days she had no pain. Today, Anita does not need pain medications and no longer avoids crowded roads, playing tennis, or family time. She practices mindfulness daily. When she notices her pain triggers, she practices responding instead of reacting. Anita lives a better life with more ease and less pain.

Spotlight: Meditation

Meditation lowers heart rate, respiratory rate, and the stress response. In a randomized controlled study, meditation decreased knee pain and arthritis pain while lowering stress levels and improving function, mood, and quality of life. This free practice works better than many medications.

There are many forms of meditation, but one of the simplest is a meditation focusing on your breath. You can do it anywhere — on a train ride into work, before a meal, in your parked car after work, after a walk, or at bedtime. An easy way to start a five-minute meditation practice is to link the new practice to a specific, daily habit at the same time each day. For example, you might resolve to meditate for five minutes in bed after you set your alarm clock.

To begin, pick a quiet, comfortable spot and sit with your

back comfortably supported and feet on the floor. You may want to set a timer so that your mind is free to focus on breathing. Your eyes may be closed or in a downward gaze. Focus on your breath, taking deep breaths in and out. It is helpful to rest your hand on your belly and feel your belly rise (expand) as you inhale and fall as you exhale. Many people enjoy silently repeating a mantra — a particular word, phrase, or sound — in conjunction with the breath. One of my favorites is "So calm." Repeat "so" in your mind as you slowly inhale, pause for a count of three, and then repeat "calm" as you slowly exhale. Give it a try. After five minutes or longer, assess how you feel. Does your mind feel clearer? Are your muscles more relaxed?

There are many types of meditation, including guided imagery and breath-focused practices. Guided imagery often involves listening to a recording or working with an instructor who guides you to focus on positive images. One example (for people who enjoy the beach) is to close your eyes and visualize being at the beach — seeing the blue ocean waves, breathing and tasting the salty air, pausing, hearing the water splashing over and over again, and noticing the sand on your feet. The practice involves mindfully engaging in a positive experience to trigger the relaxation response. Many online recordings of guided imagery are available.

Another fun technique flashes us back to our teenage years: taking three deep, dramatic, angsty sighs! Give it a try — take a gut-wrenching, slow, and gigantic inhale followed by a loud, slower, and dramatic exhale. Feel free to add an adolescent eye roll. This works well to trigger the relaxation response before or after facing a stressor.

Spotlight: Breathing Techniques

With practice, breathing exercises enable us to step back from stress and save us from a panicky or irrational survival reaction.

The US Navy teaches a technique called tactical breathing to counter the fight-or-flight response during a stressful situation. It involves inhaling for a count of four, pausing for a count of four, and exhaling for a count of four. This pattern is performed three to five times. But making the exhalation longer can enhance the relaxation response. The 4-7-8 breathing method taught by Dr. Andrew Weil is an example. Sit upright with a downward gaze or closed eyes. Ideally, keep your tongue in contact with the top of your mouth, behind your teeth, throughout the exercise. Next, breathe in through the nose for a count of four, hold the breath for a count of seven, and breathe out through the mouth for a count of eight. Repeat three more times. If these counts feel too long, you can modify them, but it is important to pause after inhaling and to exhale more slowly than you inhale. Try practicing this technique every day. If you feel your stress rising in reaction to a nasty email or a rude comment, use this exercise to break the stress cycle before you respond. It helps reduce tension, lower anxiety, control anger, handle cravings, and ease us into sleep. Four breaths to a less painful life. Ready to try?

Another well-established form of meditation is called progressive muscle relaxation. In this method, muscle groups throughout the body are intentionally tensed and then relaxed, usually working from the toes to the top of the head. Sometimes consciously feeling the tension in our muscles allows us to savor the release. We can then recall that sensation and remind ourselves to relax when we feel our muscles tensing involuntarily.

Below are samples of helpful meditations and other pain-reducing techniques. Additional recommendations are posted on my website, www.salonisharmamd.com.

MINDFULNESS AND MEDITATION TECHNIQUES FOR PAIN RELIEF
- mindfulness practice during daily activities (walking, eating, listening)

- breathing practices (e.g., 4-7-8 breathing, tactical, teenage sighs)
- meditation with a mantra (see more examples below)
- progressive muscle relaxation
- guided imagery

In addition, some movement practices, such as yoga, tai chi, and qigong, teach awareness of the breath and can also have a meditative component.

MANTRAS FOR MEDITATION

- **Stress meditation:** *This is stress. Stress is a part of life. May I find some relief. May I be kind to myself.*
- **Loving-kindness:** *May I live with ease. May I be safe and healthy. May I be happy. May you live with ease. May you be safe and healthy. May you be happy.*
- **Calm trust:** *I am confident. I am certain. I am calm.*
- **So calm:** *So* (inhale, pause for a count of three) *calm* (exhale).

Shifting Your Pain Mindset

If you suffer from chronic pain, you may have started telling yourself a pain story: *I will never feel better. I will always have this much pain. Nothing has worked to stop it, so why bother?* Patients share these fears and frustrations with me every day. They are natural thoughts, in part because of our mind's negativity bias. We tend to focus on and recall negative information more readily than positive information. For example, an image of Aunt Edna writhing in pain from sciatica sticks in our minds a lot more than the memory of two other aunts hiking the Appalachian Trail despite sciatica. When we envision our future, we see Aunt Edna, not the other two aunts. This negativity bias may be a survival instinct meant to ingrain negative experiences in our memory so that we do not repeat them. Whatever the reason it exists, in combination with pain, it may prevent us from taking action and getting better.

Our beliefs, thoughts, and feelings shape our pain mindset. Our mindset determines our actions and results. Ready for the best news? We have the power to take back control, improve that mindset, and feel better.

Pain beliefs and feelings are based on memories, experiences, cultural norms, childhood experiences, and observation of family members and acquaintances. They contribute to our pain mindset, which in turn influences our behaviors and our results. If we believe that we are destined to suffer, then we will. If we believe that we have the power to relieve our suffering (with support and guidance), then we will.

What are your beliefs about suffering? Why do you want to feel better (what are your big goals)? How have your beliefs and feelings helped or hindered you in adding Relief-5R microboosts to your day? Consider the questions below to see how your pain beliefs may be affecting your recovery.

- Do you deserve to have less pain and suffering?
- Do you believe you can have less pain and suffering?
- Do you believe small steps can help you suffer less?
- Do you believe you can add microboosts to your life?
- Do you believe you can feel better?
- Do you truly want to feel better?

If the answer to all these questions is not a strong, resounding yes, or if you want to expedite pain relief, then let's start optimizing your pain mindset and building pain resilience. We decide whether we are going to suffer. Studies have shown that recently hospitalized people who believe they are being punished or abandoned by God have a significantly higher risk of death.

Their belief directly affects their health, pain level, suffering, and lifespan. Conversely, if you believe you can get better and suffer less (regardless of your religious beliefs), then your thoughts and feelings will support this pain belief. They will motivate you to change your behaviors in ways that combat painful inflammation. According to an article in *Science*, "The experience of pain arises from both physiological and psychological factors, including one's beliefs and expectations."

It is time for you to decide your pain future. The focus of your attention will influence that outcome. If you focus on feeling bad, suffering, and picturing endless pain, then these thoughts will lead you to more stress, inflammation, and pain. Your thoughts influence your actions: if you believe that your situation is hopeless, you will do nothing to try to change it.

If, on the other hand, you focus on feeling better, doing more, and having less pain, then you will take action to lower your pain and live better, and this will become your reality. Our feelings exist on a spectrum, and nobody expects us to live without ever feeling fear or anger, or even without grieving for (but not dwelling on) the ideal, pain-free life we had envisioned for ourselves. But our focus and the majority of our feelings, thoughts, and actions must help us rise if we want to feel better. These are what will help free us from suffering. Our mindset determines whether we will rise above the pain and break free (figure 6.4). I know which way I want to go.

A "rise" mindset and coping strategies lessen pain and eliminate suffering. Coping strategies are the way we handle pain. Rise strategies include a positive outlook, hope for the future, and rich social interactions. Sink strategies include a negative outlook, poor social interactions, and catastrophizing (focusing on the worst possible result). They hamper relief and leave us in pain longer. Chronic pain studies have shown that better coping responses correlate with a quicker recovery and greater resilience.

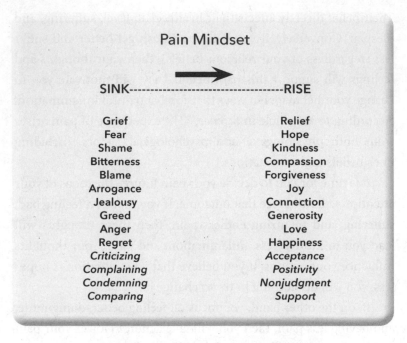

Figure 6.4. Sink or rise pain mindset.

Stress-induced feelings and beliefs can distort rational thinking and impair our coping skills. The term *cognitive distortion*
refers to thought patterns arising in the survival brain that are
irrational and harmful. For many people, pain brings cognitive
distortions to the forefront. The list below includes pain examples
and the kind of sink thinking that keeps us suffering and stuck.
Refresh microboosts help us move beyond these and promote recovery.

COMMON PAIN-RELATED COGNITIVE DISTORTIONS
- **Catastrophizing:** Always dwelling on the worst-case sce-
  nario
- **Personalizing:** Blaming yourself for pain

- **Polarized thinking:** Believing pain is an all-or-nothing situation; if you cannot live entirely pain-free, you are doomed to constant pain
- **Mind reading:** Assuming you already know what other people are thinking about you; for example, *they don't think my pain is real*
- **Overgeneralizing:** Deciding that all events will lead to same outcome based on one experience; for example, *physical therapy did not help in the past, so it cannot help now*
- **Mental filtering:** Focusing on the negatives and ignoring the positives

To combat the negativity bias, established pain beliefs and thoughts, and pain-induced cognitive distortions, we must actively redirect our thinking. Even without pain, research has shown that it takes three positive thoughts or comments to cancel out the impact of one negative one. With practice, we can train ourselves to respond to a negative pain thought with three positive thoughts:

> **Negative thought:** I will always have this much pain.
> **Positive thoughts:**
> Some times of the day, I have less pain.
> I have many options for pain control, including microboosts.
> Orthopaedic pain is common. Other people conquer it, and so will I.

Reframing your thinking in this way resets your outlook so that you can take pain-relieving action instead of spiraling into inaction and hopelessness. A positive outlook is part of a rise response and leads to less pain and suffering. When faced with ongoing pain or a painful flare, your response influences your recovery.

Managing Pain and Eliminating Suffering

A negative mindset in the face of chronic pain is not our fault; but it is something that only we can change. An important first step is to acknowledge our pain and associated emotions. If we reject or deny them, or attribute them to other causes, we suffer. Once we acknowledge pain and the feelings associated with it, then we can practice ways to manage and reduce them using mindfulness, meditation, breathing techniques, and other microboosts.

Everybody has pain at some point in their lives, and some of us experience it daily. Pain is a part of life, but suffering — the emotional and mental burden of pain coupled with a loss of our life narrative — does not have to be. Our response to pain determines whether we suffer. As part of a rise mindset, we must separate our identity from pain. Pain does not get to define us, just as a person who has diabetes is more than a "diabetic." Similarly, we cannot let one disappointment define our day. Pain may disrupt our day, but it does not get to *be* our day.

There are many well-established meditation tools to disrupt negative thinking patterns, but pain comes with a special set of challenges. Sometimes, we need help preventing pain from taking over. A mindfulness tool for compassion popularized by Tara Brach is RAIN (recognize, allow, investigate, and nurture). I have created a modified mindfulness tool for pain awareness and response: PAIN (pause, accept, inquire, now decide).

The first way to prevent painful suffering is to pause and accept that this is what you are feeling in the moment. This allows you to recognize what you are feeling instead of fighting it. Trying to ignore or resist your pain-related feelings is futile — they will continue, grow stronger, or resurface in another way. They are natural and should be addressed instead of suppressed.

Pause and Accept: *I am anxious or scared about my back pain. I worry that this pain is going to get worse.*

After pausing and acknowledging the feeling,

Inquire gently: *What thought is feeding this feeling?*
What belief is driving this feeling?

Inquiring means zooming out and reflecting on the triggers.

Now decide: *Do I need to act? Are there steps I can take to keep the pain from getting worse or disrupting an activity?*

Deciding brings your thoughts and actions back within your control.

For example, if you are worried about going out to dinner because you fear your back pain will flare up, *pause and accept* your worry, and notice that this thought may already have triggered tightness in your back. *Inquire* about what beliefs and feelings are driving this pain worry: *My pain always ruins everything. It always hurts more when I try to do something fun. I am doomed to pain and should skip going out.*

Once you have *paused*, *accepted*, and *inquired* about your pain beliefs, feelings, and thought patterns, *now decide* what you can do to ensure a better outcome. Would a mindfulness or meditation exercise before dinner lower your stress, inflammation, and pain? Would this exercise or an ATO help right now to prevent a flare? Are there practical steps you can take to help ensure a better outcome, like requesting a table near the door to minimize walking? Would sitting through dinner be less painful if you took a lumbar pillow with you? Can you wear a pain-relief patch or take medication (cleared by your physician) to minimize your pain and help you enjoy the evening? Once you've thought about your options, determine what steps to take. Remember, thoughts and feelings do not define or control you. Use the PAIN tool, an ATO, or a quick breathing exercise to pull yourself out of the sink mindset and feel better.

The Placebo and Nocebo Effects

You may have heard of the placebo effect. Our minds cause our bodies to respond to a fake treatment with a positive, healing response — proof of the mind-body unity. Positive expectations for pain relief from a fake treatment, such as sugar pills, results in less pain. A review of more than thirty-nine studies focused on back and joint surgeries found that 78 percent of people who underwent a sham surgery (in which an incision was made but no surgical intervention was done) reported significantly less pain afterward.

The placebo effect is a real, complex phenomenon that we can use to our benefit. Studies show that the placebo effect triggers the release of natural painkillers (endogenous opioids), as well as the feel-good neurotransmitters dopamine and serotonin. If we believe and expect that a proven pain strategy or microboost such as a mindfulness practice will help our pain, then it is more likely to trigger the release of natural painkillers, reinforcing our belief. Unlike pain medications, addictive substances, and psychiatric medications, our mind does this for free, and without side effects. The placebo effect changes the body's biochemistry and promotes healing. While I do not recommend eating sugar pills to reduce pain, I do advocate believing that true pain relief is possible. Committing to and trying Relief-5R strategies correlates with better pain outcomes.

The opposite is true as well: negative beliefs trigger physiological responses that can increase pain and make us feel worse. Although it is less widely discussed, the *nocebo effect* has a more powerful effect on the experience of pain. Expecting pain to continue or worsen despite the use of a relief strategy is likely to negate the effect of the strategy. It is part of the "sink" mindset of pessimism, anxiety, and catastrophizing. Nocebo suggestions (such as "That never works," or "It didn't work for my friend, so it won't work for me") trigger anticipatory anxiety, which spikes cortisol (increasing stress and painful inflammation) and blocks natural painkillers and reward pathways in the brain. Studies have confirmed that this outlook sets us up for failure (figure 6.5).

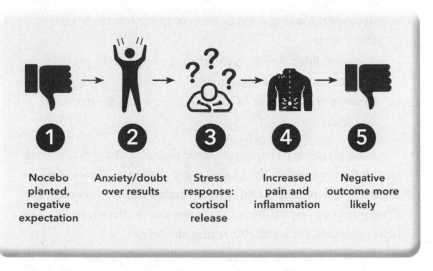

1	2	3	4	5
Nocebo planted, negative expectation	Anxiety/doubt over results	Stress response: cortisol release	Increased pain and inflammation	Negative outcome more likely

Figure 6.5. The nocebo outlook.

Study after study has proved that positive pain expectations activate opioid pain-relieving pathways and decrease anxiety, depression, and stress levels. Positive expectations act as a pain medication, antidepressant, and relaxant in one. Pain expectations and beliefs truly affect pain relief. We have the power to lessen pain and stop suffering with a change in mindset.

Resilience

Resilience is the capacity to handle a stressful setback and not only survive but also learn and grow from it. It does not mean having an instant answer to every problem or coping with everything on your own. (We will examine the power of social relationships to alleviate or worsen pain in chapter 7, "Relate.") Resilient people recognize a stressor, develop a plan to cope with it, obtain the needed tools, use them, and overcome the stressor. Resilience helps us return to a state of balance (homeostasis). Three components of resilience are recovery, sustainability, and growth.

- **Recovery:** Making a quick and complete return to a balanced state
- **Sustainability:** Ability to continue supportive, positive activities and social encounters
- **Growth:** Recognition of your ability to handle stressors and learn

Most people are resilient to some degree, but nobody is resilient all the time and in the face of every challenge. Developing resilience helps us handle and recover from painful stressors better. If we pump up our resilience skills, we can recover faster and be better prepared for inevitable future challenges.

Building resilience incorporates all aspects of the Relief-5R plan. It involves eating real food, adding more movement, prioritizing sleep, dedicating time to refresh, and nurturing relationships with others. There are many ways to build resilience, but it starts with self-care, strong social connections, and a sense of purpose. Little steps each day bring us closer to these goals.

Resilience rewires our brains to better handle and recover from stress. We all have the capacity to do this and lower our pain. We all encounter stressful challenges. We can rightfully acknowledge a setback as frustrating, undesired, and nerve-wracking, and then also look for a growth opportunity within it. A resilient approach results in quicker recovery from setbacks, better long-term outcomes, and less stress.

Part of the mindset shift entails visualizing setbacks as temporary and not part of our identity. Negative self-talk can lead us to identify completely with pain and adversity. But pain setbacks, challenges, and failures do not define us. Failures happen, but we ourselves are not failures. We may have knee pain, but that pain does not define us and our destiny.

One way to build self-confidence and resilience is to pause and remember the challenges we have conquered in the past. These successes remind us that we will survive and can thrive. This type of thinking pulls us out of survival-brain mode.

We are often prone to envision the worst-case outcome to a challenging situation. Preparing for the worst can be natural and helpful to consider, but it is not healthy to dwell on. Instead, try pausing, accepting the situation, and then focusing on developing a plan. If your plans and dreams have been derailed by injury or chronic pain, it is okay to feel sad and disappointed, as long as you do not get stuck in perpetual mourning. The goal is acceptance and moving forward with a plan. Studies demonstrate that people with a positive outlook recover from physical and psychological stressors more quickly and fully. This is resilience. Resilient people have an optimistic yet realistic attitude toward the future. They remember and are proud of overcoming other challenges. This thinking aligns with the rise mindset of having compassion for ourselves and others.

With practice, resilient thinking becomes automatic, and we suffer less, confident that we can handle and overcome challenges. When we apply this mindset to handling chronic pain, the key is acknowledging and accepting the pain situation, then recognizing that we can improve it. If we are running on overdrive with nonstop stress, poor eating and sleep habits, and no ATOs, then the burden of pain or any additional setback can feel like the final straw. When we feel overloaded, we lose sight of the fact that we have the power to choose our path forward.

The ingredients for increasing resilience are embedded in the Relief-5R program. They include improving our thought process and outlining our life purpose and big goals (table 6.1). There will be more on defining guiding life goals in chapter 7, "Relate."

Table 6.1. Increasing resilience with the Relief-5R plan.

SELF-CARE
Refuel: Eat real, unprocessed, and colorful food.
Revitalize: Add more daily movement and standing.
Recharge: Prioritize restorative sleep.
Refresh: Take adult time-outs.

SOCIAL CONNECTIONS
Relate: Nurture positive relationships.
Relate: Show gratitude.
Relate: Be part of a community.
Relate: Take time to connect every day.

PURPOSE
Refresh: Pause and reflect.
Refresh: List realistic goals and break them down into small, daily steps.
Refresh: Strive toward realistic goals.
Relate: Define your passion.
Relate: Find meaningful ways to pursue your passion.

FOCUS AND CONCENTRATION
Refresh: Engage mindfully in activities.
Refresh: Engage in meditation, breathing, and similar practices.
Refresh: Dedicate screen-free times.
Refresh: Do one thing at a time, without multitasking.

REWIRING YOUR BRAIN
Refresh: View challenges as opportunities to pause and change.
Refresh: Cultivate optimism; have hope for a better future.
Refresh: Brainstorm ways to address problems.
Refresh: Visualize yourself achieving your goals.
Refresh: Be kind to yourself, especially when you make mistakes.
Refresh: Acknowledge and track your progress and achievements.
Relate: Compare yourself only to who you were yesterday and nobody else.

Letting Go of Worry

In the Disney movie *Frozen*, Elsa sings a song called "Let It Go." This advice holds for many things in life, including anger, fear, and worry. Here we will focus on worry. It is important to be prepared for the future and consider all outcomes, good and bad. But constantly replaying negative scenarios in your mind does not help you overcome them. Instead, it paralyzes you. It activates survival-brain mode and amplifies stress, anxiety, inflammation, and pain.

If you are worried about something and there is something you can do to secure a better outcome, then do it. If there is nothing you can do, then release the worry. If public speaking makes you anxious but you have to make a presentation, repeatedly envisioning yourself freezing, stuttering, and failing does not help. Ask yourself if what you are doing is helpful. If the answer is no, then let it go. Instead, focus on simple ways to improve the outcome by breaking the problem down into smaller, controllable steps. Write the presentation out and begin practicing it in the mirror or in front of friends. Improve your speaking skills with a public speaking phone app or join an in-person or online club. You might rehearse your presentation in front of a trusted friend to get some feedback about your delivery and content.

Similarly, if you are worried about your knee pain flaring up at a graduation party, instead of repeatedly envisioning yourself limping around or missing the event, pause and ask, Is this helpful? (Hint: the answer is no.) Then, ask, What *would* be helpful? You could plan to wear a knee brace, use a topical pain-relief patch, or take a seat cushion for better knee alignment. You could skip the fancy shoes and wear the supportive ones. Before the party, you could take medication and make sure you rest your leg so you can last longer. You could ask a family member to reserve a seat for you close to the door or take something small to prop up your leg. Breaking the problem into little steps and tackling these makes the best possible outcome more probable. Always remember that you have faced and conquered other challenges in the past, and despite the stressful feeling, you will survive this pain challenge and learn from it.

Sometimes we need help pausing and avoiding a negative thought spiral. In addition to the PAIN thought tool, physical tools are helpful, too. There are many practical ways to pause, regroup, and take on a challenge. It can be helpful to "peck" at the problem with the PECC plan: *pause, engage* in the present, *check* your thoughts, and *create* a plan, using some of the tactics outlined in table 6.2.

Table 6.2. Practical ways to PECC at challenges.

PAUSE
Accept the moment and your initial response.
Try not to assume the worst-case outcome.
Think of a time when you conquered another challenge.
Write down three things you are grateful for right now.
Envision a source of joy (a person, place, or thing).
Take three deep breaths with a long inhale, pause, and longer exhale.
Sigh three times, slowly, fully, loudly.
Consider a stress or loving-kindness meditation.

ENGAGE
Look outside or at a picture of a pet or loved one.
Focus on a scent: a flower, a scented oil or candle, or fresh air.
Focus on the taste and texture of a piece of gum, a smooth cashew, or a refreshing mint.
Run your fingers over a seashell, fidget toy, fabric, or your fingernails.
Focus on sounds around you: rain pattering, birds chirping, or a fan buzzing.
Listen to your favorite song.
Connect with a friend, colleague, or loved one.

CHECK
Monitor your self-talk: Is this how you would talk to a friend in the same situation?
For repeated worries, ask, *Is this helpful?*
Convert worry to action: Ask, *What can I do that would be helpful?*
Take a break: Is there time for a full or miniature adult time-out?

CREATE
Brainstorm solutions.
Ask, *Is this a chance to learn or do something new?*
Develop a plan.
Break the plan into smaller steps.
Start working on the first step.

A useful tool for engaging in the present is a collection of *refresh anchors*, physical objects and sensory cues that remind us of something joyful, helping to keep us out of a negative thought spiral. Refresh anchors may include a scented candle or aromatherapy oil, dried fruit or nuts whose flavor and texture we can savor, a recording of a favorite song, a seashell with an appealing texture, or a favorite picture. Engaging the senses in a pleasant way evokes positive feelings and thoughts that better prepare us to face the challenge. It helps us stop the painful stress spiral and reconnect with the present. As in the popular television show *Grey's Anatomy*, sometimes you have to dance it out.

For decades, we have known that environmental design matters to healthcare outcomes. A soothing environment facilitates the PECC method. Our environment includes the people in it, space, and actual design. Multiple studies have shown that patients who look at nature views, flowers, and water scenes, even for less than five minutes, have less stress and muscle spasm. Hospitalized patients with windows offering a view of nature recover faster and need less pain medication than those without a view. Nature helps us heal. If getting outside or sitting near a window with a view is not an option at your workplace or home, consider adding lush nature photographs, indoor plants, or recordings of nature sounds that you can engage with for three to five minutes when you need to lower stress and refocus.

How do we design our environment for pain relief? Consider

adding a nature focal point to every room at home and at work, if possible. Also, surround yourself with pictures of people, places, and things that bring you joy. What is the first thing you see when you wake up? What is the last thing you see before you go to sleep? Are these things helping you rise and recover? Are they promoting pain relief and prevention? At work, you may have little control over your immediate environment, so you may have to rely on your refresh anchors to provide a private environmental microboost. Let's build a physical, mental, and emotional environment that supports pain relief, healing, and well-being.

CASE STUDY

Krista, a 62-year-old woman, lived with constant back pain that had worsened over the previous two years. She had been diagnosed with degenerative disc disease and had been taking daily NSAIDs and nightly muscle relaxers. She lived with tightness, aches, spasms, and constant, grinding pain. The medications enabled her to go to work and manage basic activities like walking, dressing, cooking, cleaning, and sleeping, but she still experienced pain. During her initial visit, we discussed conventional medical treatments. We touched on the Relief-5R program and scheduled an appointment for a deeper dive after her upcoming vacation.

At her next visit, she reported, in shock, that all of her pain had "magically" disappeared for the duration of her five-day beach trip. She returned on a Saturday and did minor things like unpacking her suitcase. On Sunday afternoon, she started thinking about her Monday morning meetings and felt her back tighten up. After her first Monday meeting, her pain returned in force.

Krista had discovered on her own that stress was a major driver of her pain, and perhaps the only one. Just to be clear, her disc degeneration was still present: it did not miraculously heal during her vacation and then reappear. But the painful inflammation disappeared while she was on vacation and returned when she returned to a stressful environment. Simply thinking about work on Sunday re-ignited her pain.

Although changing jobs might have been the ideal solution, it was not a realistic option for Krista at the time. Instead we focused on identifying stress-relieving micro-boosts she could employ throughout the day, including mindfulness techniques, breathing exercises, refresh anchors, and adult time-outs. We reviewed her schedule and added time around her more stressful activities for using her refresh anchors and quick microboosts. Her job remains chaotic, but the stress no longer consumes her or causes pain. If she feels pain creeping in, she uses a microboost to calm it. Krista no longer needs daily NSAIDs and muscle relaxers. She lives a better life with less stress, less pain, less medication, and more ease.

Mindset Jump Start

Our ultimate goal is to change our beliefs and feelings about pain. However, changing our mindset takes time and does not happen without setbacks, when we are vulnerable to negative beliefs, feelings, and thoughts. Sometimes we have to start with action rather than beliefs. Even if we do not feel like taking action, we have to get up and move, take a walk, or use the PAIN tool, a refresh anchor, or another microboost to keep ourselves from spiraling down into pain.

This approach rests on linking microboosts to daily habits. We can quickly start building a rise mindset for less pain and a better life by taking action.

❖

We cannot avoid painful challenges, but we can learn to better cope with stressors, lower painful inflammation, and improve our mindset so that pain does not rule our lives. We do not have to suffer. Taking time to refresh and cultivate resilience empowers us to handle stressors with acceptance, compassion, and strength. Life's challenges are like waves in an ocean: some are big and some are small, but they never stop flowing. Each wave tests our balance and resilience. We can learn to ride the ups and downs. The big wipeouts can sink us or teach us how to rise with grace. Cultivating a response that can override a survival-brain reaction brings back control. Building resilience starts with microboosts.

Too often, we disappoint ourselves if we do not quickly overcome a painful setback. We may also feel resentment, believing that other people have easier paths. This mindset burdens us with self-doubt, anxiety, anger, sadness, and more pain. Accepting our present situation frees us to forge a path forward, transforming grief to relief, and rage to courage. We often believe the path to overcoming a painful setback is straightforward, like climbing a ladder, but this is not reality. Facing painful challenges is more like rock climbing — thinking through each step and working around obstacles at our own pace and in our own unique way (figure 6.6).

Each step prepares us to better handle the next step and brings us closer to our goals. Sometimes we may feel like we're sidestepping or even moving backward, but each step represents progress. These steps include building resilience, committing to self-care, and coming up with practical ways to handle painful challenges. A shift in our mindset from resistance and fear to acceptance and hope reduces stress, pain, and suffering. Instead of worrying about what we do not have or cannot do, what if we focus on what we *do* have and what we *can* do? Let's refresh and build our capacity to handle painful stress with a tangible, custom pain relief plan (figure 6.7).

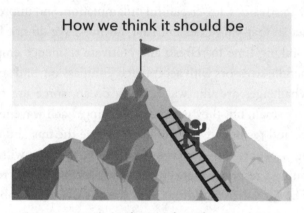

A simple, straight path

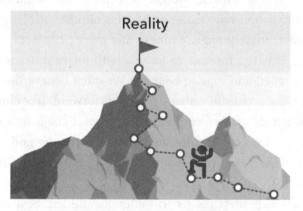

Step-by-step, small achievements

Figure 6.6. Facing pain challenges.

SET FOR SUCCESS: REFRESH

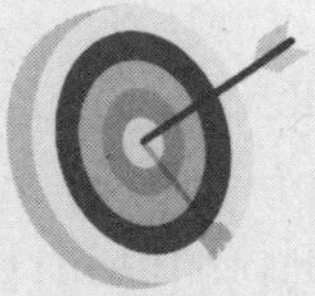

R   REMOVE BARRIERS
- **Intention:** Try a mindfulness application.
- **Microboost:** *I will download a free app now, try it, and put it on my first home screen.*

E   EYE LEVEL
- **Intention:** Make a refresh anchor bag.
- **Microboost:** *I will gather a collection of anchors and a small bag on my counter throughout the day and assemble it after dinner.*

L   LINK TO A SPECIFIC ACTIVITY
- **Intention:** Complete a daily adult time-out.
- **Microboost:** *After I brush my teeth, I will take a ten-minute ATO in bed.*

I   "I" DECLARATION
- **Intention:** Be more present and minimize multi-tasking.
- **Microboost:** *Say aloud, "I will not look at screens at dinner." Write down, "No screens at dinner." I will put screens in a shoebox at dinner time.*

E   ENCOURAGE PROGRESS BY TRACKING
- **Intention:** Keep track of my Refresh activities.
- **Microboost:** *I will note each daily ATO on a calendar or app.*

F   FEEL BETTER!

Figure 6.7. Relief-5R method for creating customized Refresh microboosts.

Next Steps

1. Review your big goal — what you want to achieve (or prevent) by making changes.
2. From the list below, identify two microboosts that fit your life and will help you progress toward your goal.
3. Turn these microboosts into a custom Relief-5R plan with specific action steps, following the examples below.
4. Envision your big goals and know you are on your way to achieving them.
5. Feel better!

MICROBOOSTS LEVEL 1

*   Pick an adult time-out and schedule it on your calendar like a daily appointment.
*   Try five minutes of meditation focusing on your breath, with or without a silent repeated phrase, consider: "So" (inhale, pause for a count of three) "calm" (exhale).
*   Practice four cycles of 4-7-8 breathing daily or when faced with a painful stressor.
*   Pick one routine activity to practice mindfully every day, such as walking, eating, or listening.
*   Try a guided mindfulness exercise (using a phone app or website) every morning or every night as part of your bedtime relaxation routine.
*   Make a collection of refresh anchors. Put them in a bag and keep it with you to use before a work meeting, doctor's appointment, or other times you feel you may get caught in a stress or pain thought spiral.
*   Think about tasks you often end up juggling and make a plan for dealing with them one at a time as much as possible.

- When faced with a stressful challenge, peck at it with the PECC plan (pause, engage, check, create).
- Create a to-do list that schedules specific amounts of time for tasks along with transitions, relaxation, and human connection.
- Identify a habitual negative thought and reframe it in a positive way. Ask, Is this helpful? Then ask, What *would* be helpful? Add more placebo, skip the nocebo.
- Even if you do not feel like taking action, get up and move, walk, or do a mindfulness activity to break free from a negative thought spiral.
- Make a list of previous painful and stressful challenges you have overcome. Refer to it when you feel trapped to see proof that you can overcome this painful challenge, too.
- When you find yourself sinking into a painful sink thought spiral, use the PAIN tool (pause, accept, inquire, now decide).

MICROBOOSTS LEVEL 2

- Pick a pain or stress meditation to use and repeat to yourself when things get rough, for example, a loving-kindness meditation: *May I live with ease. May I be safe and healthy. May I be happy.*
- Include nature scenes, plants, and nature sounds in your environment.
- Pick an activity you enjoy and plan how and when to incorporate it into your daily routine.

CUSTOM RELIEF PLAN: EXAMPLES

- *I will listen to music for ten minutes at 6 p.m. in my car.*
- *I will practice mindfulness for ten minutes at 7:30 a.m. in my family room.*

- *I will walk, screen-free, for ten minutes at 3 p.m. in the park.*
- *I will create a refresh anchor bag.*
- *I will add a photograph of my favorite nature scene or vacation to a room where I spend a great deal of time at home or work.*

CHAPTER 7

Relate

We need to more deeply appreciate the relationship between loneliness, social connection, and physical and emotional health.

— Vivek H. Murthy, MD

Myth: Poor relationships do not affect orthopaedic pain.

Fact: Loneliness and stressful relationships worsen orthopaedic pain.

Relief-5R: Improving relationships and responses is part of a true pain solution.

With resilience, we can recover, sustain, and grow in the face of painful challenges. The cornerstones of pain resilience are relationships with others and ourselves. Regular and positive interactions with others support our mental and emotional well-being. Conversely, if pain derails these interactions, preventing us from regularly seeing friends and loved ones, we suffer more and may sink deeper into pain. Positive interactions promote pain tolerance and recovery.

Social Relationships

Humans are hard-wired to belong. For much of our evolutionary history, being part of a tribe or group was vital to our physical survival. It protected us from predators and natural elements. It allowed us to build living areas, farm, and hunt. It enabled us to protect our young ones, the sick, and the weak. It gave us a role and a sense of purpose. Today, being part of a community is still important to our healthspan and lifespan. It still gives us a role and sense of purpose. A sense of belonging triggers a release of feel-good chemicals in our brain that promote healing and pain relief. In fact, without social connections our health falters. Isolation or feeling lonely can be as deadly as smoking fifteen cigarettes a day! It chips away at our health and pain tolerance. There is a reason why solitary confinement is used as one of the ultimate punishments. Its influence extends beyond the confinement period. A study published in the *American Journal of Public Health* found that solitary confinement correlates with more depression, anxiety, loss of identity, further social isolation, and pain than are found in general prison populations. A 2020 study demonstrated that those in solitary confinement had more orthopaedic pain. While these are extreme examples, they highlight the harm of being or feeling socially isolated.

At some level, we are all aware of the power of physical or perceived isolation and loneliness. The physical distancing, lockdowns, remote working, and quarantining mandated by the Covid-19 pandemic increased feelings of loneliness for many people. Studies found that only three weeks into stay-at-home orders, feelings of loneliness, depression, and suicidal thoughts skyrocketed. We are truly dependent on social interactions to thrive and survive.

Thankfully, we have the ability to improve our pain resilience through social connection. Another pandemic study found resilience greater in those who felt more socially supported, spent more time outdoors, exercised more, and slept better. These findings confirm the importance of the Relief-5R pillars.

The most meaningful social relationships involve close family, close friends, a romantic partner, volunteer work, and religious groups, but they may include neighbors and coworkers as well. While we may consider work, school, or volunteer relationships less significant than family connections and close friendships, these are often the contexts in which we interact most frequently with people. Positive daily human connections, even casual ones, help us feel better and flourish.

Feeling isolated activates the stress response, raises cortisol, increases inflammation, increases defensiveness, and decreases sleep quality. Poor relationships and loneliness are stressors just like poor food, lack of exercise, and disrupted sleep.

Feeling socially isolated impairs daily functioning. A study published in the *Archives of Internal Medicine* found that lonely people are more likely to develop difficulties in activities like dressing, eating, and walking. Lack of support results in a greater risk of developing musculoskeletal problems. A systematic review found that poor social support could be used as a predictor of chronic low back pain. In addition, social isolation results in weight gain and may contribute to the development of inflammatory conditions such as diabetes as well as mental health issues.

The impact of poor social interactions on the pain mindset cannot be overlooked either. Toxic social interactions feed a negative mindset of comparison, complaints, and criticisms. If there is room for us to distance ourselves from people who practice this kind of mindset at work, in the community, or at home, it can help our own mindset. This type of thinking is often contagious and does not support pain relief. If it is not possible to distance ourselves from such people, we can practice an extra refresh microboost after interacting with them, such as mindful breathing or an ATO. Once again, the mind and body work as one unit to feed or quell pain and inflammation.

Thankfully, the data show that we can not only reduce our pain level with better social connections but also lower our risk of future musculoskeletal pain. Social relationships have a direct relationship with pain and inflammation. Studies demonstrate that good social relationships correlate with lower inflammatory markers, specifically high-sensitivity CRP and interleukins. A review study of forty-one articles found that social support and integration correlated with lower inflammation levels.

Strong social connections are vital to our health, well-being, and pain control (table 7.1).

Table 7.1. Social connections and well-being.

RISKS ASSOCIATED WITH POOR SOCIAL CONNECTIONS	BENEFITS OF GOOD SOCIAL CONNECTIONS
More pain	Less pain
More inflammation	Less inflammation
Obesity	Less numbing, addictive eating
Antisocial behavior	More inclination to support and connect with others
Impaired focus, problem-solving, and coping	Better focus, problem-solving, and coping ability
Depression and anxiety	Less depression and anxiety, lower suicide risk
Alcohol and drug abuse	Less numbing behaviors
Diabetes	Lower diabetes risk
Heart disease	Lower risk of heart disease

Dementia	Lower risk of dementia
Stroke	Greater overall health
Headaches	
Stomach problems	
Premature aging	Healthy aging
Shorter healthspan	Longer healthspan
Shorter lifespan	Longer lifespan

Not All Social Connections Are Equal

There is truth in the adage that we are the average of the people we spend the most time with. Our environment, including the people around us, affects our phenotype. Our family, friends, neighbors, coworkers, and other connections model what we come to believe is "normal" in all aspects of life, from behavior, weight, social status, finances, eating habits, and sleep patterns to resilience, pain tolerance, and pain coping. A thirty-year study of over twelve thousand people found that a person's risk of becoming obese increased by 57 percent if a friend became obese, by 40 percent if a sibling became obese, and by 37 percent if their spouse became obese. Investigating smoking cessation, the same study found that a spouse quitting smoking lowered the other person's likelihood of smoking by 67 percent, a friend quitting lowered the risk by 36 percent, and a sibling quitting lowered the risk by 25 percent. The people in our lives influence the behaviors that determine our well-being, and we influence them in turn. If we hang out with a negative, unhealthy crowd, it should be no surprise if our well-being declines and pain increases. The converse holds true as well: a mindful group with a positive mindset supports pain resilience and improvements in our own well-being — including our behaviors, attitudes, and lifestyle choices — which help improve the well-being of our loved ones and community. This is the kind of domino effect we want!

Happy people cluster. A twenty-year study of more than 4,500 people found that people surrounded by happy people are more likely to be happy in the future. A happy friend increases your chance of feeling happy by 25 percent. Unfortunately, the same study found that unhappy clusters also exist and may be more powerful.

The Pain-Relationship Connection

Why do we find ourselves stuck thinking about pain? Why do we dwell on each aspect of the hurt? Why does it pervade our life? It is not our fault. In chapter 6 we examined the negativity bias and saw that although it may have evolved to protect us from life-threatening dangers, it does not always benefit us in the modern world. Focusing on negative beliefs, feelings, and thoughts about pain hampers recovery. These thoughts shrink our world down to nothing but pain and allow it to rule us. This mindset limits our ability to think clearly, solve problems, and connect with others. It feeds the poison of social comparison (figure 7.1). We can overcome this tendency by building our own pain resilience and protecting ourselves with supportive interactions.

Part of the pain solution entails using tools like the PAIN thought-processing tool, mindfulness, and gratitude (as introduced in previous chapters), which enable us to shift our focus from resenting and mourning the things we do not have to recognizing and appreciating what we do have. Gratitude also prevents us from making toxic social comparisons. It gets us out of our own heads and allows us to connect with and support others. And connection, in turn, makes us feel better.

A hallmark of negativity is a set of behaviors known as the Four Cs: criticizing, complaining, condemning (judging), and

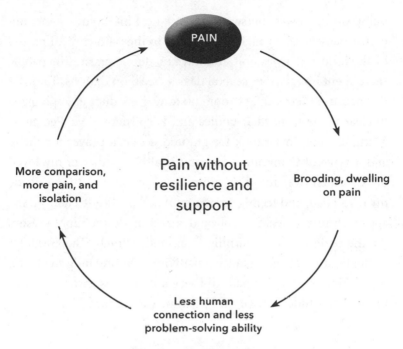

Figure 7.1. Pain cycle.

comparing. If we surround ourselves with company that makes these behaviors habitual, we are likely to find ourselves in a negative mindset that leads to more pain. We waste precious brainpower judging others as good or bad instead of accepting them as they are. We sacrifice awareness of the present to dwell on the past or worry about the future. We miss joyful moments. The more we practice the Four Cs, the more we reinforce them, and the more we feed painful inflammation and inhibit our capacity for healing and growth.

Sometimes we cannot avoid exposure to the negative attitudes of others, and it takes an effort of awareness to trigger feelings of gratitude and break free. When I was in my medical training, it was easy to let the toxic people around me weigh me down. There was always a bitter resident, physician, or nurse ready to dump on the lowest person in the medical hierarchy — me. But on my daily walk through the hospital to the pain clinic, I passed by the kidney dialysis unit. It always made me pause. The people there spent hours a day, several days a week, on dialysis. They did this because their kidneys could no longer produce enough urine to clear waste from their bodies and keep them alive. Peeing — a simple thing that I took for granted. I said a prayer for them, and a wave of thankfulness for my health and that of my loved ones washed over me. This moment of pausing, getting outside my own head, and feeling compassion and gratitude changed my approach to my negative colleagues and made me more present for the patients I was learning from and helping. The antidotes to the Four Cs are acceptance, positivity, avoiding judgment, and supporting others. The path to these antidotes is through mindfulness, gratitude, service, and learning (figure 7.2).

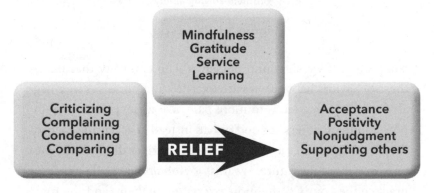

Figure 7.2. Relate mindset path to pain relief.

Maintaining a positive mindset and relationships does not mean we should never talk about our troubles. Venting at work, recapping difficult situations, and bonding over a struggle build relationships. If the discussion focuses on investigation, understanding, and uplifting (others and ourselves), then it is beneficial.

Since the behavior of those around us influences our wellness, pain, and inflammation, it can benefit us if we find a *mentor* — someone who radiates an attitude of positivity, acceptance, nonjudgment, and helping others. This person inspires us to grow, improve, heal, serve, and show gratitude; to think better, act better, and be better. They rise above and elevate themselves and others. This person may be somebody you know, like a kind family member, friendly coworker, or philanthropist, or it may be a famous person or bygone figure such as Mahatma Gandhi, Mother Teresa, or Fred Rogers. It may even be a fictional character, such as the coach Ted Lasso from the television show *Ted Lasso* or Leslie Knope from *Parks and Recreation*. If you can interact with your mentor directly, so much the better; but if you cannot, then think about what they would do in your situation. What steps would they take to feel better? What advice would they give you? Would they let fatigue or time stop them from achieving their goals?

In addition to a mentor, another tool is simply asking yourself, *Is it kind?* You can ask this of all your actions. Is it kind to myself to stay up late looking at social media and be exhausted tomorrow? Is it kind to judge that person as bad based on one statement? Asking this question helps us focus on caring for ourselves and others. It frees us from the burden of condemning, criticizing, complaining, and comparing, enabling us to focus on being better and getting better. If you practice this kind of thinking, you may soon notice a change in the way people interact with you, too. They may reflect your positive attitude back to you. You can create your own happy cluster — a healthy ecosystem in which you support others and they support you.

Some people may feel married to pain and suffering. For them, thinking about their own wellness is not a strong enough motivation to change; but considering the well-being of loved ones, friends, and community may be inspiring. Do we want to help build a happy cluster or an unhappy cluster? What gifts can we offer to those around us? We can only give what we have. If we are filled with suffering and negativity, then those are the only things we can share. Focusing on these thoughts lets them grow. If we want to uplift others, we must start by uplifting ourselves.

Well-being refers to a state of health and happiness. A positive mindset helps us handle pain and limit suffering, and it is a critical component of well-being. The World Health Organization's constitution defines health as "a state of complete physical, mental and social well-being and not merely an absence of disease or infirmity." This definition lies at the heart of pain control. We cannot truly relieve pain and end suffering without addressing the mental, emotional, and social aspects of pain as well as the physical ones. The Centers for Disease Control and Prevention (CDC) elaborates the definition of well-being to include what we think and feel about our lives in addition to mental and physical health.

WELL-BEING: CDC DEFINITION AND ASSOCIATIONS
- mind-and-body approach to preventing disease and promoting health
- quality relationships
- positive emotions with fewer negative emotions
- life satisfaction
- realizing potential and productivity
- social connections

The CDC notes that addressing the well-being of both mind and body is linked to lower rates of illness and injury as well as to quicker recoveries. A sense of well-being includes an understanding of our relationship with others and ourselves — our beliefs, our self-talk, and our purpose.

Self-Talk

We have explored the importance of our beliefs about pain, but the way we talk to ourselves matters, too. Unfortunately, the negativity bias and pain-induced survival-mode thinking tend to foster negative self-talk. If we are constantly berating ourselves for every misstep, we nurture feelings of anger, fear, shame, and grief, which feed rather than quell our pain. We want to extend compassion, forgiveness, and kindness to ourselves as well as others. The question "Is it kind?" applies as much to our self-talk as to our thoughts and actions concerning others.

One way to check our self-talk is to think about it from another person's perspective. How do we talk to ourselves when we make a mistake? How would we respond to a child or loved one if they made the same mistake? Probably not so critically. We would trade the nastiness for loving-kindness and concern for their well-being. Can we extend that compassion to ourselves? If it is hard to break a pattern of critical, negative self-talk, one remedy is to reach out to our mentor or a supportive person. They will listen, remind us of the good things we have accomplished, and maybe help us find a path forward. Microboosts such as mindfulness and gratitude exercises can also help pull us out of a spiral of negative self-talk.

We also need to stop listening to other voices that falsely tell us we are not measuring up. The media, retail industry, and sometimes well-intentioned friends and family members promote the fallacy that the path to better well-being depends on a certain job, a perfect relationship, a bottomless bank account, or excessive attention to our appearance. This is untrue. Research has shown that higher levels of well-being are cultivated by nurturing supportive relationships; spending time with loved ones; feeling gratitude, optimism, and mindfulness; savoring the moment; developing strong coping skills; and pursuing a lifelong goal (figure 7.3).

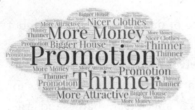 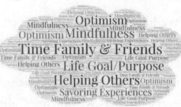

Figure 7.3. What people often think builds well-being (left) vs. what actually does.

Service and Prosocial Acts

Some of the best things we can do for ourselves are not about us at all. When we are feeling down and off track, one of the easiest ways to feel better about ourselves and the situation is to help others. This is called a *prosocial act* and does not necessarily mean committing to curing cancer or caring for people with leprosy. You could contribute to your community by tutoring local children, organizing a litter pickup, or linking your community to a project at work. You might promote volunteer work at your company or employ one of your skills for the greater good. If baking is your "jam," you might consider delivering homemade baked goods to a rehabilitation center or nursing home once a week. This could expand to running an online cooking class or organizing a book drive for the center. A goal of this kind, involving service to others, may not relieve all your pain, but it eases suffering. It feeds repair and growth.

Social connection and service do not have to be onerous, time-consuming acts. They can be little acts of kindness that we can feel good about when we reflect on them at the end of the day. At work, you might listen to an elderly widow describe her recently deceased husband for an extra three minutes. You might volunteer for a few hours at a community center or hospital or other organization. You might simply indulge a cantankerous neighbor complaining about his old kidney stone, offer a smile to a woman new to the area, or hold the door open for somebody at the doctor's office.

These little gestures of caring elevate mood-boosting and pain-relieving pathways. One four-week study compared the well-being of people assigned to complete weekly self-focused activities, such as treating themselves to a special dessert, and another group assigned to perform weekly prosocial acts, such as helping a neighbor. The prosocial group felt more positive emotions and an improved sense of well-being, while the self-focused group reported no improvement. Two weeks after the study ended, the prosocial group still reported more positive emotions and higher levels of well-being. Helping others truly helps us, too.

Even for people with limited energy and mobility, there are many opportunities for prosocial acts. One of my friends puts his spare change into a jar every day and donates the money to a different charity every month. He even invites other friends to vote for the charity online. Another easy act of caring is to buy a few extra canned goods or granola bars at the grocery store and donate them to a local food bank. Boosting others boosts us, too, even through small acts like making sure that traffic stops for a child waiting at a crosswalk or saying a genuine thank-you to a store clerk. If you feel yourself getting stuck in negative thinking and need a quick microboost, try remembering something kind you did for someone else. Consider banking some prosocial acts for a painful, rainy day!

Another form of healthy engagement is a creative project. Humans are made to create and to find joy in the process as well as the product. You might choose painting, cooking, writing, woodwork, designing, scrapbooking, photography, or inventing a new exercise routine. Some people direct their creativity into their jobs by developing new workflows, presentations, and articles — whatever rings your bell. This invigorates your mind and frees you from pain. Of course, acute pain and severe pain flare-ups require immediate attention, but once the pain has been evaluated by a physician and settled down to a more tolerable level, come back to your project and refocus your mind on all you have to give and all that you are lucky to have. Remember, positive thinking reduces pain and inflammation. To take it a step further, positive thinking with a purpose quells pain and restores joy.

Part of the personal benefit of service and creative projects comes from reflecting on how your efforts benefit others. If three people are baking cookies for a charity bake sale, they may all view the activity differently. The first person says, "I am baking cookies." The second person says, "I am helping raise money for the charity." The third person says, "I am helping kids with disabilities get better educational tools." The second and third people view their actions as serving a bigger purpose and helping others. Knowing that they are making a difference in the world triggers the release of feel-good, pain-fighting substances in their brains. Similarly, three physical therapists working with a patient with leg weakness after a stroke might have different perspectives on their work. The first therapist says, "I am teaching her leg exercises." The second says, "I am helping her walk better." The third says, "We are getting her ready to walk at her daughter's wedding." They are all teaching the same exercises, but only the third therapist views their work as part of their own and the patient's bigger purpose. This therapist feels more invested and experiences more gratification as the patient improves. Helping others helps ourselves.

Are you embracing your passions? Even if you have to modify your activities, are you practicing your passion every day? Our goal is to contribute to our community in a way that gives us more joy, supports a rise mindset, and stops suffering. A positive relationship with others and ourselves helps us repair and grow.

Cultivating Awe and Gratitude

In addition to practices like adult time-outs, mindfulness, meditation, gratitude, forest bathing, and breathing exercises, other ways to promote well-being include cultivating awe and gratitude.

Awe is a sense of wonder and feeling part of something bigger than yourself. Feeling awe gives us perspective and stops us from painful brooding. A 2020 study analyzed two groups of people who walked outside daily for fifteen minutes and took selfie pictures during their walks. One group was instructed to look for sources of awe; the other was instructed simply to walk. The people taking "awe walks" reported more positive emotions and joy during the walk, and less stress afterward, than the other group. Interestingly, the smiles of the awe walkers, as shown in their selfies, grew in intensity over the multiweek study. Even more telling, their faces became smaller in the selfie pictures. Their focus shifted from themselves to appreciating what was around them. This fantastic microboost intentionally shifts our attention outward instead of inward. As we have already seen, another microboost, gratitude, improves well-being, reduces stress, and lowers painful inflammation. A gratitude practice starts and ends our day on the right note. It may sound nebulous and overpromoted, but it truly makes us feel better. As with all microboosts, pick and customize the method so it works best for you.

GRATITUDE MICROBOOSTS

- **Gratitude journal:** Each night, list three things you are grateful for in phone notes or on paper. One way to enliven this practice is to list one person, one place, and one thing you are grateful for (I call this "the concrete three").

- **Gratitude trigger:** Carry an object you can look at, such as a memento of a special place, that triggers gratitude.
- **Shared gratitude:** Create a ritual of daily sharing, perhaps asking everyone at the dinner table to share something they are grateful for, or sharing with family or friends over the phone.
- **Focused gratitude:** Every day, tell a loved one something about them that you are grateful for (a quality, or something they did); can be a two-way practice.
- **Expressing gratitude:** Every day, send a text, email, or note thanking somebody.

A gratitude practice that boosts social connection, like shared, focused, or expressed gratitude, is doubly beneficial.

❖

Authenticity, meaning, connection, and clarity about our path help us better handle painful challenges. We suffer less. A positive mindset combined with a meaningful life goal can empower us, helping us fight the negativity bias and painful inflammation. We all have pain and stressors, but how we handle them determines whether pain and suffering engulf our lives. The worksheet below helps us identify ways we can boost well-being and stop suffering (figure 7.4).

What is your life goal? What matters most to you? Who matters most to you? A life goal might be improving the community by organizing a program that engages elders or beautifies the neighborhood, being a role model for children, improving access to education, or revolutionizing the healthcare industry. It must

RELATE WELL-BEING

Life goal

_____
_____
_____

Belief and self-talk

_____
_____
_____

Gratitude

_____
_____

Prosocial acts

_____
_____
_____

Joy and awe

_____
_____
_____

Creativity

_____
_____
_____

Figure 7.4. Relate well-being worksheet.

be an activity that is meaningful to you and serves others — in your neighborhood or across the world.

Let's use the following questions to help complete the worksheet.

- Do you believe that you can do it? What is your plan for facing doubts and staying positive so that you can rise above pain and pursue your goal? This may include talking with your mentor and supportive friends, and recalling previous accomplishments.
- What are you grateful for? How do you practice gratitude daily?
- What are your prosocial activities? Prosocial acts, big and small, give us perspective and gratitude for what we have.
- Do you find joy and awe daily? Where and how can you add more of these pain-fighting elixirs to your day and environment?
- Do you spend some time weekly or daily creating in a way that brings you joy? This could be cooking new meals, sewing, woodworking, painting, making music, or writing, to name just a few possibilities.

Your life goal may combine many of the relate well-being factors! Let's raise our outlook and lower painful inflammation.

Integrating our favorite microboosts into our day or week helps us recover from painful challenges, reduce stress, gain perspective, and focus on our life goal. It is a framework for feeling better, improving well-being, and reducing suffering with a tangible, customized Relief-5R plan (figure 7.5).

Next Steps

1. Review your big goal — what you want to achieve (or prevent) by making changes.

SET FOR SUCCESS: RELATE

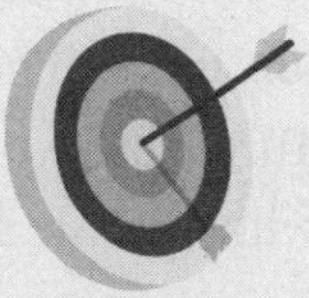

R REMOVE BARRIERS
- **Intention:** Consider an awe walk.
- **Microboost:** *I will set a daily phone alarm after work for an awe walk.*

E EYE LEVEL
- **Intention:** Spend more time on the creative activity that brings me joy.
- **Microboost:** *I will place my sketchbook and pencils in front of my computer.*

L LINK TO A SPECIFIC ACTIVITY
- **Intention:** Connect with my friends and family more often.
- **Microboost:** *After dinner, I will call or text a loved one.*

I "I" DECLARATION
- **Intention:** Show more compassion to others and myself.
- **Microboost:** *I will ask, "Is it kind?" I will write down, "Is it kind?" and tape it to my bathroom mirror. I will put an "Is it kind?" note on the home screen of my phone and pause to consider it when feeling stressed.*

E ENCOURAGE PROGRESS BY TRACKING
- **Intention:** Keep track of my progress in cultivating gratitude and relationships.
- **Microboost:** *I will keep a gratitude notebook.*

F FEEL BETTER!

Figure 7.5. Relief-5R method for creating customized Relate microboosts.

2. From the list below, identify two microboosts that fit your life and will help you progress toward your goal.

3. Turn these microboosts into a custom Relief-5R plan with specific action steps, following the examples below.

4. Envision your big goals and know you are on your way to achieving them.

5. Feel better!

MICROBOOSTS LEVEL 1

- Pause and practice a quick mindfulness or breathing exercise when dealing with unavoidable toxic people.

- Practice compassion, mindfulness, and gratitude when talking to yourself and others.

- In all your actions toward yourself or others, ask, *Is it kind?*

- Make time to perform prosocial activities weekly or daily, and recall these activities when you're feeling down.

- Get involved with people in your neighborhood, community, spiritual group, or workplace who are energetic and uplifting to be around.

- Find a mentor to emulate and to help you.

- Read new books or learn new skills to sharpen your brain and gain perspective.

- Create things that bring you and others joy: art, music, meals, tools, blankets, and books!

- Get motivated by thinking about the way your positive mindset can trigger happiness in those around you.

- Define your life goal — what drives you, gives you purpose, and brings you and others joy and relief.

- Remember to boost yourself with adult time-outs, mindfulness, meditation, forest bathing, and breathing exercises.

- Schedule a daily fifteen-minute awe walk.
- Track gratitude daily to feel better: consider a gratitude journal, shared gratitude, focused gratitude, the concrete three, a gratitude trigger, or gratitude expression.

Microboosts Level 2

- What activities bring you joy? List them and compare them to your daily schedule. Schedule fifteen to thirty minutes a day to do an activity that brings you joy.
- What people bring you joy? Make time weekly to spend time with somebody who brings you joy (in person, if possible, or by video chat).
- Send a daily text or make a daily call to check in on loved ones.

Custom Relief Plan: Examples

- *I will spend twenty minutes after dinner knitting.*
- *I will spend twenty minutes after dinner reading a fun book or magazine.*
- *I will text a different friend or loved one every night after dinner for a week.*
- *I will smile at every person I see today at the store, work, and home.*
- *I will volunteer at my community center this Saturday.*

CHAPTER 8

The Path

*It's impossible to predict the future… [but] once you design
something, it changes the future that is possible.*

— BILL BURNETT AND DAVE EVANS

Designing a future with less pain — a better life — starts with
our choices now. Those choices address our pain, stressors,
and challenges in a resilient way. Pain and inflammation are signals that physical, emotional, and/or mental stressors require our
attention: they are red flags. If we ignore them, they grow stronger
and manifest themselves in other painful ways. How we respond
determines our success. If we react with fear, resistance, and pessimism, we suffer more. Pain and suffering may consume our
lives and leave us hopeless or dependent on temporary, artificial
forms of relief. But if we acknowledge the messages and thought-
fully respond with the Relief-5R plan, we quell pain and stop suffering. We build pain resilience and prevent pain. We thrive, not
just survive.

Unfortunately, the conventional healthcare system, with its
focus on treating disease, manages pain poorly. It views pain

as a condition separate from the entire person and located in a specific part of the body. It lacks a plan for increasing pain resilience, preventing pain, or improving well-being. The Relief-5R plan is a different solution that brings pain relief, wellness, and ease (figure 8.1).

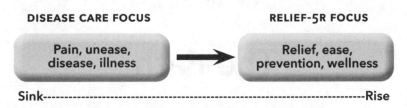

Figure 8.1. Relief-5R approach.

We know that lasting pain relief entails treating the whole person — mind and body. The Relief-5R plan homes in on the bodily aspects of pain relief though the Refuel, Revitalize, and Recharge pillars, and the mind aspects through the Refresh and Relate pillars. Our big goal motivates us to take action, and concrete microboosts create a path forward. For some people, the best way to start is simply by adding one microboost a day from each pillar (table 8.1).

Table 8.1 Sample microboosts.

REFUEL	REVITALIZE	RECHARGE	REFRESH	RELATE
Replace meat with plant protein once a week on the same day.	Add more steps to your day by parking farther away at the store and walking, or taking a longer walking route.	Create a relaxation routine.	Take an adult time-out.	Save the words, "Is it kind?" to your phone's home screen.

REFUEL	REVITALIZE	RECHARGE	REFRESH	RELATE
Place healthier snacks like nuts, apples, hummus, and veggies front and center in your kitchen.	Take short movement breaks at work and at home.	Prioritize your sleep schedule.	Try a mindfulness activity.	Consult a mentor when feeling stuck or doubtful.
Avoid added sugar.	Walk outside with a friend.	Build a sleep cave.	Pause, accept, inquire, now decide.	Complete a prosocial act daily: smile at a stranger, hold the door open for someone, take a few extra minutes to listen to a child's or neighbor's story.
Try circadian eating.	Do a routine of spine stretches daily.	Turn off screens thirty minutes before bed.	Make a refresh anchors bag.	Dedicate fifteen to twenty minutes a day to creating or learning something new.

It is critical to customize microboosts in a way that links them to your daily activities. Willpower fails, but habit and simplicity prevail. The RELIEF guide reminds us how to integrate microboosts into our existing routine so that they become healthy new habits.

R   Remove barriers
E   Eye level
L   Link to a specific activity
I   "I" declaration
E   Encourage progress by tracking
F   Feel better!

It is important to keep it simple when adding daily microboosts. If they seem difficult or are not well integrated into your daily routine, it may be difficult to stick with them.

Our pain mindset matters, too. At some point, we all have pain, but whether we suffer depends on how we approach pain, stress, and challenges (table 8.2). This can be the difference between relief and stagnation.

Table 8.2 Pain mindset.

SINK	RISE
I can't feel better.	I can feel better.
I don't believe I will feel better.	I will feel better.
I don't deserve to feel better.	I deserve to feel better.
This is too hard. I am failing.	This will be challenging, but I can do it.
The pain will never get better.	The pain will get better.
I am doomed to suffer.	I am not doomed to suffer.
My whole life will be painful.	My whole life does not have to be painful.
There's no point in trying.	I have a healing intention.

Getting a Jump Start on Pain Relief

Some people benefit from a more structured approach to forming new habits. A fourteen-day pain-relief jump start gets us moving. Review the microboosts for each pillar in the Relief-5R plan (at the end of chapters 3–7) and pick two microboosts from each pillar. For the first week, commit to adding one microboost from each pillar to your day. The following week, add a second microboost, so that you are doing two microboosts from each pillar daily. A worksheet can help you plan your jump start and track your progress (figure 8.2). Write down each of your chosen microboosts and check a box on the worksheet for each day you accomplish it.

A helpful way to evaluate the effectiveness of this approach is to track your pain and, more important, your daily activity and joy levels, before, during, and after the fourteen-day jumpstart. Start tracking one week before you begin the jump start and continue for a week afterward. You may do this on your phone, a calendar, a journal, or the back side of your worksheet. We cannot expect months or years of pain and inflammation to vanish in fourteen days, but we can look for some positive changes in our pain, activity, and joy levels.

If you are not seeing progress, and your pain has already been evaluated by your physician, then you may need to try different microboosts or enact them at different times of the day. Commitment and dedication are critical to get results. Inevitably, there will be setbacks and tough days. When these happen, the Refresh tools will help you pause, give yourself grace, and start again.

Congratulations on getting started — may this book guide you on a simple, drug-free path to true pain relief and prevention.

With love and gratitude,
SALONI SHARMA, MD

PAIN-RELIEF JUMP-START WORKSHEET

	REFUEL	REVITALIZE	RECHARGE	REFRESH	RELATE
WEEK 1	MICROBOOST:	MICROBOOST:	MICROBOOST:	MICROBOOST:	MICROBOOST:
	S M T W T F S	S M T W T F S	S M T W T F S	S M T W T F S	S M T W T F S
WEEK 2	MICROBOOST 1:	MICROBOOST 1:	MICROBOOST 1:	MICROBOOST 1:	MICROBOOST 1:
	S M T W T F S	S M T W T F S	S M T W T F S	S M T W T F S	S M T W T F S
	MICROBOOST 2:	MICROBOOST 2:	MICROBOOST 2:	MICROBOOST 2:	MICROBOOST 2:
	S M T W T F S	S M T W T F S	S M T W T F S	S M T W T F S	S M T W T F S

Figure 8.2. Fourteen-day jump-start worksheet.

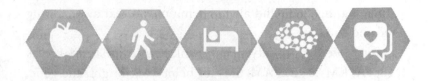

Acknowledgments

Thank you to all the healthcare workers caring for people in a system that often forgets them. You are my heroes and inspire me to do more.

Thank you to these spectacular and motivating physician groups: LGA, EWP, LMP, PMG, PPMG, FPE, WPW, SAWPNA, DPM, KevinMD, WP, and WPPM.

A big thank you to Dr. Weil and the Andrew Weil Center for Integrative Medicine teachers, staff, and fellows for advocating for whole-person healthcare and encouraging this book.

Thanks to everyone on the New World Library team who helped me through this process. A special thanks to the thoughtful and patient Georgia Hughes.

Thank you to my agent, Jill Marsal, for giving me a chance.

A heartfelt thank you to my communities — blessed to go through life's ups and downs together: the ROI community, TE community, and Pittsburgh community.

A special thank you to my medical school friends, especially SP and SS, who believed in this book and always go the extra mile for their patients, family, and friends.

Thank you to the PMRD (MD, GT, KH, NA, VV, PO) for

supporting this book and always being only a text away during good and bad times.

For more than twenty years, thank you to the F&M Ladies (MB, PA, KM, SP, DE, AM, SM) for being your bright, energetic, and opinionated selves, and encouraging me to do this.

Thank you to my newest community, BMML (SH, AJ, ALP, CD, DGM, DG, JL, MM, PG, YB, ZS), for advising me and striving to juggle motherhood, culture, friendship, and professional life together.

Thank you to all of my teachers and mentors who are shining examples of making the world a better place, from Shady Side to Hershey Medical Center to Thomas Jefferson University (especially SW, VG, and MF). An extra thanks to the Jeff triangle (RA, JT), the OIHC team, JS, and JV.

Thank you to MD/S, a talented physician and author, who supported me through this process and is my kindred spirit, hype woman, creative genius (though she denies it), and forever chief.

A warm thank you to the Sharma family (near and far), Wells family, and Jaitley family for their continuous love and support. I am eternally grateful for Mom, Dad, MS, and PS for always being there and filling my life with love and light.

A giant hug, a handful of tickles, and two kisses to MW and LW. Thank you for calling me an author long before this book and reminding me to look for joy in every moment.

Thank you to MW for believing in me and giving me the time and space to write this book in between piano lessons, work trips, baseball practice, birthday parties, and a pandemic. I love you and what we are becoming.

List of Illustrations

Notes

Introduction

p. 1   *an estimated 80 percent of Americans experience back pain*: Devon I. Rubin, "Epidemiology and Risk Factors for Spine Pain," *Neurologic Clinics* 25, no. 2 (2007): 353–71.

Chapter 1: The Pain Problem

p. 7   *The way modern medicine operates*: Mark Hyman, *The Blood Sugar Solution: The Ultrahealthy Program for Losing Weight, Preventing Disease, and Feeling Great Now!* (New York: Little, Brown Spark, 2012).

p. 9   *More than 54 percent of Americans report musculoskeletal pain*: T. C. Clarke, R. L. Nahin, P. M. Barnes, and B. J. Stussman, *Use of Complementary Health Approaches for Musculoskeletal Pain Disorders among Adults: United States, 2012*. National Health Statistics Report no. 98 (2016), 1–8.

p. 9   *A crisis of addiction*: National Institute on Drug Abuse, "Overdose Death Rates," www.drugabuse.gov/drug-topics/trends-statistics/overdose-death-rates.

p. 9   *More than ten thousand lives a year*: Marie R. Griffin, "Epidemiology of Nonsteroidal Anti-inflammatory Drug–Associated Gastrointestinal Injury," *American Journal of Medicine* 104, no. 3 (1998): 23S–29S.

p. 9   *Low back pain alone causes more disability*: Stephen S. Lim, Theo

Vos, Abraham D. Flaxman, Goodarz Danaei, Kenji Shibuya, Heather Adair-Rohani, Markus Amann, et al., "A Comparative Risk Assessment of Burden of Disease and Injury Attributable to 67 Risk Factors and Risk Factor Clusters in 21 Regions, 1990–2010: A Systematic Analysis for the Global Burden of Disease Study 2010," *Lancet* 380, no. 9859 (2012): 2224–60.

p. 11   *One in five adult Americans report pain every day*: R. Jason Yong, Peter M. Mullins, and Neil Bhattacharyya, "Prevalence of Chronic Pain among Adults in the United States," *Pain* (April 2, 2021).

p. 13   *More than 68 percent of Americans receive at least one prescription*: Wenjun Zhong, Hilal Maradit-Kremers, Jennifer L. St Sauver, Barbara P. Yawn, Jon O. Ebbert, Véronique L. Roger, Debra J. Jacobson, Michaela E. McGree, Scott M. Brue, and Walter A. Rocca, "Age and Sex Patterns of Drug Prescribing in a Defined American Population," *Mayo Clinic Proceedings*, 88, no. 7 (2013): 697–707.

p. 13   *Almost 40 percent take more than five prescription medications*: Elizabeth D. Kantor, Colin D. Rehm, Jennifer S. Haas, Andrew T. Chan, and Edward L. Giovannucci, "Trends in Prescription Drug Use among Adults in the United States from 1999–2012," *JAMA* 314, no. 17 (2015): 1818–30.

p. 13   *Diet and other lifestyle changes could prevent 80 percent of inflammatory conditions*: World Health Organization, *Preventing Chronic Diseases: A Vital Investment*, 2005, www.who.int/chp/chronic_disease_report /full_report.pdf.

p. 15   *Maintaining a healthy weight, being physically active, not smoking, and limiting alcohol intake increased healthy years*: Solja T. Nyberg, Archana Singh-Manoux, Jaana Pentti, Ida E. H. Madsen, Severine Sabia, Lars Alfredsson, Jakob B. Bjorner, et al., "Association of Healthy Lifestyle with Years Lived without Major Chronic Diseases," *JAMA Internal Medicine* 180, no. 5 (2020): 760–68.

Chapter 2: The Relief-5R Plan

p. 19   *In many cases, the outcome you want*: James Clear, "3-2-1: Starting from Zero, and How to Choose What to Work On," June 24, 2021, https://jamesclear.com/3-2-1/june-24-2021.

p. 20   *More than 60 million Americans have had a recent bout of back pain*:

Georgetown University, Health Policy Institute, Chronic Back Pain, https://hpi.georgetown.edu/backpain/#.

p. 24   *Excess body fat... adds to physical stress*: Noriyuki Ouchi, Jennifer L. Parker, Jesse J. Lugus, and Kenneth Walsh, "Adipokines in Inflammation and Metabolic Disease," *Nature Reviews Immunology* 11, no. 2 (2011): 85–97.

p. 25   *Belly fat... consists of active cells that produce inflammatory molecules*: Hye Soon Park, Jung Yul Park, and Rina Yu, "Relationship of Obesity and Visceral Adiposity with Serum Concentrations of CRP, TNF-α and IL-6," *Diabetes Research and Clinical Practice* 69, no. 1 (2005): 29–35.

p. 25   *This can lead to early back arthritis... and other conditions*: Binwu Sheng, Chaoling Feng, Donglan Zhang, Hugh Spitler, and Lu Shi, "Associations between Obesity and Spinal Diseases: A Medical Expenditure Panel Study Analysis," *International Journal of Environmental Research and Public Health* 14, no. 2 (2017): 183; Rebecca Wilson Zingg and Richard Kendall, "Obesity, Vascular Disease, and Lumbar Disk Degeneration: Associations of Comorbidities in Low Back Pain," *PM&R* 9, no. 4 (2017): 398–402.

p. 29   *NSAIDs... block the production of cytokines*: L. Gallelli, O. Galasso, D. Falcone, S. Southworth, M. Greco, V. Ventura, P. Romualdi, et al., "The Effects of Nonsteroidal Anti-inflammatory Drugs on Clinical Outcomes, Synovial Fluid Cytokine Concentration and Signal Transduction Pathways in Knee Osteoarthritis: A Randomized Open Label Trial," *Osteoarthritis and Cartilage* 21, no. 9 (2013): 1400–1408.

p. 30   *91 percent of patients in the United States*: Haytham M. A. Kaafarani, Kelsey Han, Mohamad El-Moheb, Napaporn Kongkaewpaisan, Zhenyi Jia, Majed W. El-Hechi, Suzanne van Wijck, et al., "Opioids after Surgery in the United States versus the Rest of the World: The International Patterns of Opioid Prescribing (iPOP) Multicenter Study," *Annals of Surgery* 272, no. 6 (2020): 879–86.

p. 31   *Long-term use of opioids increases painful inflammation*: Catherine M. Cahill and Anna M. W. Taylor, "Neuroinflammation: A Co-occurring Phenomenon Linking Chronic Pain and Opioid Dependence," *Current Opinion in Behavioral Sciences* 13 (2017): 171–77.

p. 31   *A higher rate of fractures*: Fumin Ping, Ying Wang, Jing Wang, Jie Chen, Wenxian Zhang, Hua Zhi, and Yugang Liu, "Opioids Increase Hip Fracture Risk: A Meta-analysis," *Journal of Bone and Mineral Metabolism* 35, no. 3 (2017): 289–97.

p. 31   *These hormonal changes can also lead to prediabetes*: Cassidy Vuong, Stan H. M. Van Uum, Laura E. O'Dell, Kabirullah Lutfy, and Theodore C. Friedman, "The Effects of Opioids and Opioid Analogs on Animal and Human Endocrine Systems," *Endocrine Reviews* 31, no. 1 (2010): 98–132.

p. 32   *People who take opioids over a long period*: AnGee Baldini, Michael Von Korff, and Elizabeth H. B. Lin, "A Review of Potential Adverse Effects of Long-Term Opioid Therapy: A Practitioner's Guide," *Primary Care Companion to CNS Disorders* 14, no. 3 (2012); Mark D. Sullivan, Michael Von Korff, Caleb Banta-Green, Joseph O. Merrill, and Kathleen Saunders, "Problems and Concerns of Patients Receiving Chronic Opioid Therapy for Chronic Non-cancer Pain," *PAIN* 149, no. 2 (2010): 345–53.

Chapter 3: Refuel

p. 37   *If it came from a plant, eat it*: Michael Pollan, *Food Rules: An Eater's Manual* (New York: Penguin, 2013).

p. 38   *The "sonic chip" study*: Massimiliano Zampini and Charles Spence, "The Role of Auditory Cues in Modulating the Perceived Crispness and Staleness of Potato Chips," *Journal of Sensory Studies* 19 (February 2005): 347–63.

p. 38   *Consuming real, unprocessed food reduces pain*: Ashish S. Kaushik, Larissa J. Strath, and Robert E. Sorge, "Dietary Interventions for Treatment of Chronic Pain: Oxidative Stress and Inflammation," *Pain and Therapy* 9, no. 2 (2020): 487–98.

p. 39   *Diet soda intake correlates with higher rates of inflammation*: J. A. Nettleton, P. L. Lutsey, Y. Wang, J. A. Lima, E. D. Michos, and D. R. Jacobs Jr., "Diet Soda Intake and Risk of Incident Metabolic Syndrome and Type 2 Diabetes in the Multi-ethnic Study of Atherosclerosis (MESA)," *Diabetes Care* 32, no. 4 (2009): 688–94.

p. 39   *Diet soda consumption is associated with a greater risk of kidney failure*: Casey M. Rebholz, Morgan E. Grams, Lyn M. Steffen, Deidra C. Crews, Cheryl A. M. Anderson, Lydia A. Bazzano, Josef Coresh, and Lawrence J. Appel, "Diet Soda Consumption and Risk of Incident End Stage Renal Disease," *Clinical Journal of the American Society of Nephrology* 12, no. 1 (2017): 79–86.

p. 39   *Both sugar-sweetened and diet soft drinks are linked with obesity*:
D. Ruanpeng, C. Thongprayoon, W. Cheungpasitporn, and T.
Harindhanavudhi, "Sugar and Artificially Sweetened Beverages
Linked to Obesity: A Systematic Review and Meta-analysis," *QJM:
An International Journal of Medicine* 110, no. 8 (2017): 513–20.

p. 40   *Only 1.5 percent of Americans consume an ideal diet*: Dariush
Mozaffarian, Emelia J. Benjamin, Alan S. Go, Donna K. Arnett,
Michael J. Blaha, Mary Cushman, Sandeep R. Das, et al., "Heart
Disease and Stroke Statistics — 2016 Update: A Report from the
American Heart Association," *Circulation* 133, no. 4 (2016): e38–e360.

p. 40   *The standard American diet (SAD)… breeds pain, inflammation, and
disease*: S. K. Totsch, R. Y. Meir, T. L. Quinn, S. A. Lopez, B. A. Gower,
and R. E. Sorge, "Effects of a Standard American Diet and an Anti-
inflammatory Diet in Male and Female Mice," *European Journal of
Pain* 22, no. 7 (2018): 1203–13.

p. 40   *This processed, nutrient-poor diet increases pain and inflammation*:
Stacie K. Totsch, Tammie L. Quinn, Larissa J. Strath, Laura J.
McMeekin, Rita M. Cowell, Barbara A. Gower, and Robert E. Sorge,
"The Impact of the Standard American Diet in Rats: Effects on Behav-
ior, Physiology and Recovery from Inflammatory Injury," *Scandinavian
Journal of Pain* 17, no. 1 (2017): 316–24.

p. 40   *Poor nutrition… contributes to heart disease*: World Health Organization. *Diet, Nutrition, and the Prevention of Chronic Diseases: Report of
a Joint WHO/FAO Expert Consultation* (Geneva: World Health Organization, 2003), 916.

p. 42   *Dietary recommendations from the United States Department of Agriculture (USDA)*: US Department of Agriculture, *A Brief History of USDA
Food Guides*, June 2011, available at https://myplate-prod.azureedge
.net/sites/default/files/2020-12/ABriefHistoryOfUSDAFoodGuides.pdf.

p. 43   *Switching from the SAD to a diet high in natural, unprocessed foods*:
Elizabeth Dean and Rasmus Gormsen Hansen, "Prescribing Optimal
Nutrition and Physical Activity as 'First-Line' Interventions for Best
Practice Management of Chronic Low-Grade Inflammation Associated
with Osteoarthritis: Evidence Synthesis," *Arthritis* 2012 (December 31,
2012): 560634.

p. 43   *A proinflammatory diet (like the SAD) increases feelings of distress*:
Guo-Qiang Chen, Chun-Ling Peng, Ying Lian, Bo-Wen Wang,

Peng-Yu Chen, and Gang-Pu Wang, "Association between Dietary Inflammatory Index and Mental Health: A Systematic Review and Dose-Response Meta-analysis," *Frontiers in Nutrition* 8 (2021): 662357.

p. 44   *Americans consume more sugar per person*: WorldAtlas, "Countries That Eat the Most Sugar," March 19, 2019, www.worldatlas.com /articles/top-sugar-consuming-nations-in-the-world.html.

p. 44   *Sugar activates the reward pathway in our brain*: Rudolph Spangler, Knut M. Wittkowski, Noel L. Goddard, Nicole M. Avena, Bartley G. Hoebel, and Sarah F. Leibowitz, "Opiate-Like Effects of Sugar on Gene Expression in Reward Areas of the Rat Brain," *Molecular Brain Research* 124, no. 2 (2004): 134–42.

p. 44   *Taking naltrexone*: Ileana Morales, Ileana, Olga Rodríguez-Borillo, Laura Font, and Raúl Pastor, "Effects of Naltrexone on Alcohol, Sucrose and Saccharin Binge-Like Drinking in C57BL/6J Mice: A Study with a Multiple Bottle Choice Procedure," *Behavioural Pharmacology* 31, nos. 2–3 (2020): 256–71.

p. 44   *Sugar actually changes our sense of taste*: Paul M. Wise, Laura Nattress, Linda J. Flammer, and Gary K. Beauchamp, "Reduced Dietary Intake of Simple Sugars Alters Perceived Sweet Taste Intensity but Not Perceived Pleasantness," *American Journal of Clinical Nutrition* 103, no. 1 (2016): 50–60.17.

p. 46   *The American Heart Association recommends limiting added sugars*: Rachel K. Johnson, Lawrence J. Appel, Michael Brands, Barbara V. Howard, Michael Lefevre, Robert H. Lustig, Frank Sacks, Lyn M. Steffen, and Judith Wylie-Rosett, "Dietary Sugars Intake and Cardiovascular Health: A Scientific Statement from the American Heart Association," *Circulation* 120, no. 11 (2009): 1011–20.

p. 48   *Many artificial sweeteners have been shown to alter the gut microbiome*: Francisco Javier Ruiz-Ojeda, Julio Plaza-Díaz, Maria Jose Sáez-Lara, and Angel Gil, "Effects of Sweeteners on the Gut Microbiota: A Review of Experimental Studies and Clinical Trials," *Advances in Nutrition* 10, no. 1 (2019): S31–S48.19.

p. 49   *Greater fiber consumption results in less arthritic knee pain*: Zhaoli Dai, Jingbo Niu, Yuqing Zhang, Paul Jacques, and David T Felson, "Dietary Intake of Fibre and Risk of Knee Osteoarthritis in Two US Prospective Cohorts," *Annals of the Rheumatic Diseases* 76, no. 8 (2017): 1411–19.

p. 49   *Fiber reduces the risk of prolonged pain*: Mark A. Pereira, Eilis O'Reilly,

Katarina Augustsson, Gary E. Fraser, Uri Goldbourt, Berit L. Heitmann, Goran Hallmans, et al., "Dietary Fiber and Risk of Coronary Heart Disease: A Pooled Analysis of Cohort Studies," *Archives of Internal Medicine* 164, no. 4 (2004): 370–76; Shiu-Ming Kuo, "The Interplay between Fiber and the Intestinal Microbiome in the Inflammatory Response," *Advances in Nutrition* 4, no. 1 (2013): 16–28.

p. 51   *The polyphenols found in berries*: Hui-Ying Luk, Casey Appell, Ming-Chien Chyu, Chung-Hwan Chen, Chien-Yuan Wang, Rong-Sen Yang, and Chwan-Li Shen, "Impacts of Green Tea on Joint and Skeletal Muscle Health: Prospects of Translational Nutrition," *Antioxidants* 9, no. 11 (2020): 1050.

p. 51   *An increased intake of polyphenol phytonutrients*: Chwan-Li Shen, Brenda J. Smith, Di-Fan Lo, Ming-Chien Chyu, Dale M. Dunn, Chung-Hwan Chen, and in-Sook Kwun, "Dietary Polyphenols and Mechanisms of Osteoarthritis," *Journal of Nutritional Biochemistry* 23, no. 11 (2012): 1367–77.

p. 54   *Cocoa shines as a potent pain reliever*: Martina De Feo, Antonella Paladini, Claudio Ferri, Augusto Carducci, Rita Del Pinto, Giustino Varrassi, and Davide Grassi, "Anti-inflammatory and Anti-nociceptive Effects of Cocoa: A Review on Future Perspectives in Treatment of Pain," *Pain and Therapy* 9, no. 1 (2020): 231–40.

p. 55   *Omega-3 essential fatty acids act as anti-inflammatory agents*: Marcelo Macedo Rogero and Philip C. Calder, "Obesity, Inflammation, Toll-Like Receptor 4 and Fatty Acids," *Nutrients* 10, no. 4 (2018): 432.

p. 55   *Omega-3 supplementation decreased pain levels*: Young-Ho Lee, Sang-Cheol Bae, and Gwan-Gyu Song, "Omega-3 Polyunsaturated Fatty Acids and the Treatment of Rheumatoid Arthritis: A Meta-analysis," *Archives of Medical Research* 43, no. 5 (2012): 356–62.

p. 55   *Omega-3 fatty acid supplementation decreases spinal disc injury*: Zachary NaPier, Linda E. A. Kanim, Yasaman Arabi, Khosrowdad Salehi, Barry Sears, Mary Perry, Sang Kim, Dmitriy Sheyn, Hyun W. Bae, and Juliane D. Glaeser, "Omega-3 Fatty Acid Supplementation Reduces Intervertebral Disc Degeneration," *Medical Science Monitor: International Medical Journal of Experimental and Clinical Research* 25 (2019): 9531.

p. 55   *Omega-3 fatty acids... may also decrease muscle atrophy*: Chris McGlory, Philip C. Calder, and Everson A. Nunes, "The Influence of

Omega-3 Fatty Acids on Skeletal Muscle Protein Turnover in Health, Disuse, and Disease," *Frontiers in Nutrition* 6 (2019): 144.

p. 55   *Omega-3 supplements with antioxidant vitamins enhance physical health*: Pinelopi S. Stavrinou, Eleni Andreou, George Aphamis, Marios Pantzaris, Melina Ioannou, Ioannis S Patrikios, and Christoforos D Giannaki, "The Effects of a 6-Month High Dose Omega-3 and Omega-6 Polyunsaturated Fatty Acids and Antioxidant Vitamins Supplementation on Cognitive Function and Functional Capacity in Older Adults with Mild Cognitive Impairment," *Nutrients* 12, no. 2 (2020): 325.

p. 56   *Supplementing with omega-3 reduces pain*: Robert J. Goldberg and Joel Katz, "A Meta-analysis of the Analgesic Effects of Omega-3 Polyunsaturated Fatty Acid Supplementation for Inflammatory Joint Pain," *Pain* 129, no. 1–2 (2007): 210–23.

p. 56   *Omega-3 supplementation resulted in pain reduction*: Joseph Charles Maroon and Jeffrey W. Bost, "ω-3 Fatty Acids (Fish Oil) as an Anti-inflammatory: An Alternative to Nonsteroidal Anti-Inflammatory Drugs for Discogenic Pain," *Surgical Neurology* 65, no. 4 (2006): 326–31.

p. 57   *SPMs reduce inflammation*: Nan Chiang and Charles N Serhan, "Specialized Pro-resolving Mediator Network: An Update on Production and Actions," *Essays in Biochemistry* 64, no. 3 (2020): 443–62.

p. 58   *The presence of SPMs in the knee joint fluid*: Anne E. Barden, Mahin Moghaddami, Emilie Mas, Michael Phillips, Leslie G. Cleland, and Trevor A. Mori, "Specialised Pro-Resolving Mediators of Inflammation in Inflammatory Arthritis," *Prostaglandins, Leukotrienes and Essential Fatty Acids* 107 (2016): 24–29.

p. 58   *SPMs are considered by many to be the therapy of the future*: Mervin Chávez-Castillo, Ángel Ortega, Lorena Cudris-Torres, Pablo Duran, Milagros Rojas, Alexander Manzano, Bermary Garrido, et al, "Specialized Pro-resolving Lipid Mediators: The Future of Chronic Pain Therapy?," *International Journal of Molecular Sciences* 22, no. 19 (2021): 10370.

p. 58   *Decreased levels of inflammatory markers, including CRP*: Joel C. Craddock, Elizabeth P. Neale, Gregory E. Peoples, and Yasmine C. Probst, "Vegetarian-Based Dietary Patterns and Their Relation with Inflammatory and Immune Biomarkers: A Systematic Review and Meta-analysis," *Advances in Nutrition* 10, no. 3 (2019): 433–51.

p. 58   *Replacing just 3 percent of animal protein with plant protein*: Jiaqi

Huang, Linda M. Liao, Stephanie J. Weinstein, Rashmi Sinha, Barry
I. Graubard, and Demetrius Albanes, "Association between Plant and
Animal Protein Intake and Overall and Cause-Specific Mortality,"
JAMA Internal Medicine 180, no. 9 (2020): 1173–84.

p. 60   *Excessive amounts cause inflammation*: Claudio Luevano-Contreras,
and Karen Chapman-Novakofski, "Dietary Advanced Glycation End
Products and Aging," *Nutrients* 2, no. 12 (2010): 1247–65.

p. 60   *People with low back pain and lower limb pain had higher levels of
AGEs*: Tomotaka Umimura, Sumihisa Orita, Kazuhide Inage, Yasuhiro
Shiga, Satoshi Maki, Masahiro Inoue, Hideyuki Kinoshita et al,
"Percutaneously-Quantified Advanced Glycation End-Products (Ages)
Accumulation Associates with Low Back Pain and Lower Extremity
Symptoms in Middle-Aged Low Back Pain Patients," *Journal of Clinical
Neuroscience* 84 (2021): 15–22.

p. 60   *These AGEs literally age us*: Richard D. Semba, Emily J. Nicklett, and
Luigi Ferrucci, "Does Accumulation of Advanced Glycation End
Products Contribute to the Aging Phenotype?," *Journals of Gerontology
Series A: Biomedical Sciences and Medical Sciences* 65, no. 9 (2010):
963–75.

p. 61   *High dietary AGE levels cause AGE deposits in lumbar discs*: Divya
Krishnamoorthy, Robert C. Hoy, Devorah M. Natelson, Olivia M.
Torre, Damien M. Laudier, James C. Iatridis, and Svenja Illien-Jünger,
"Dietary Advanced Glycation End-Product Consumption Leads to Me-
chanical Stiffening of Murine Intervertebral Discs," *Disease Models and
Mechanisms* 11, no. 12 (2018): dmm036012.

p. 62   *Dehydration spikes pain activity*: Yuichi Ogino, Takahiro Kakeda, Koji
Nakamura, and Shigeru Saito, "Dehydration Enhances Pain-Evoked
Activation in the Human Brain Compared with Rehydration," *Anesthe-
sia and Analgesia* 118, no. 6 (2014): 1317–25.

p. 63   *Dehydration also affects brain function and mood*: Barry M. Popkin,
Kristen E. D'Anci, and Irwin H. Rosenberg, "Water, Hydration, and
Health," *Nutrition Reviews* 68, no. 8 (2010): 439–58.

p. 63   *Green tea also decreases inflammatory markers*: Luk, Appell, Chyu, et
al., "Impacts of Green Tea."

p. 66   *An unbalanced gut microbiome correlates with chronic musculoskeletal pain*: Marta Anna Szychlinska, Michelino Di Rosa, Alessandro
Castorina, Ali Mobasheri, and Giuseppe Musumeci, "A Correlation

between Intestinal Microbiota Dysbiosis and Osteoarthritis," *Heliyon* 5, no. 1 (2019): e01134; Maxim B. Freidin, Maria A. Stalteri, Philippa M. Wells, Genevieve Lachance, Andrei-Florin Baleanu, Ruth C. E. Bowyer, Alexander Kurilshikov, Alexandra Zhernakova, Claire J. Steves, and Frances M. K. Williams, "An Association between Chronic Widespread Pain and the Gut Microbiome," *Rheumatology* (2020).

p. 67   *NSAIDs change the gut microbiome composition*: Xianglu Wang, Qiang Tang, Huiqin Hou, Wanru Zhang, Mengfan Li, Danfeng Chen, Yu Gu et al., "Gut Microbiota in NSAID Enteropathy: New Insights from Inside," *Frontiers in Cellular and Infection Microbiology* 11 (2021): 572.

p. 68   *These supplements exert anti-inflammatory and antioxidant effects*: Cindy Crawford, Courtney Boyd, Charmagne F. Paat, Karin Meissner, Cindy Lentino, Lynn Teo, Kevin Berry, and Patricia Deuster, "Dietary Ingredients as an Alternative Approach for Mitigating Chronic Musculoskeletal Pain: Evidence-Based Recommendations for Practice and Research in the Military," *Pain Medicine* 20, no. 6 (2019): 1236–47; Bharat B. Aggarwal, Wei Yuan, Shiyou Li, and Subash C. Gupta, "Curcumin-Free Turmeric Exhibits Anti-inflammatory and anticancer Activities: Identification of Novel Components of Turmeric," *Molecular Nutrition and Food Research* 57, no. 9 (2013): 1529–42.

p. 69   *These spices reduce inflammatory cytokines*: Tzung-Hsun Tsai, Po-Jung Tsai, and Su-Chen Ho, "Antioxidant and Anti-inflammatory Activities of Several Commonly Used Spices," *Journal of Food Science* 70, no. 1 (2005): C93–C97;52. Monika Mueller, Stefanie Hobiger, and Alois Jungbauer, "Anti-Inflammatory Activity of Extracts from Fruits, Herbs and Spices," *Food Chemistry* 122, no. 4 (2010): 987–96.

p. 69   *Intermittent fasting… may aid in controlling pain*: Rafael de Cabo and Mark P. Mattson, "Effects of Intermittent Fasting on Health, Aging, and Disease," *New England Journal of Medicine* 381, no. 26 (2019): 2541–51.

p. 70   *People fasting for religious reasons*: Mohammad Adawi, Abdulla Watad, Stav Brown, Khadija Aazza, Hicham Aazza, Mohamed Zouhir, Kassem Sharif, et al., "Ramadan Fasting Exerts Immunomodulatory Effects: Insights from a Systematic Review," *Frontiers in Immunology* 8 (2017): 1144.

p. 70   *Periodic fasting reduces arthritic pain*: Aliki I. Venetsanopoulou, Paraskevi V. Voulgari, and Alexandros A. Drosos, "Fasting Mimicking Diets: A Literature Review of Their Impact on Inflammatory Arthritis," *Mediterranean Journal of Rheumatology* 30, no. 4 (2019).

p. 70   *Intermittent fasting increases sensitivity to opioid pain medications*:
David I. Duron, Filip Hanak, and John M. Streicher, "Daily Intermittent Fasting in Mice Enhances Morphine-Induced Antinociception
While Mitigating Reward, Tolerance, and Constipation," *Pain* 161,
no. 10 (2020): 2353–63.

p. 70   *A lower-calorie diet reduced pain*: Ana Rita Silva, Alexandra Bernardo,
João Costa, Alexandra Cardoso, Paula Santos, Maria Fernanda de
Mesquita, José Vaz Patto, Pedro Moreira, Maria Leonor Silva, and
Patrícia Padrão, "Dietary Interventions in Fibromyalgia: A Systematic
Review," *Annals of Medicine* 51, supp. 1 (2019): 2–14.

p. 70   *Intermittent fasting improves healthspan*: Iftikhar Alam, Rahmat Gul,
Joni Chong, Crystal Tze Ying Tan, Hui Xian Chin, Glenn Wong,
Radhouene Doggui, and Anis Larbi, "Recurrent Circadian Fasting
(RCF) Improves Blood Pressure, Biomarkers of Cardiometabolic Risk
and Regulates Inflammation in Men," *Journal of Translational Medicine*
17, no. 1 (2019): 1–29.

p. 70   *Intermittent fasting...has been shown time and again*: Mohammad
Bagherniya, Alexandra E. Butler, George E Barreto, and Amirhossein
Sahebka, "The Effect of Fasting or Calorie Restriction on Autophagy
Induction: A Review of the Literature," *Ageing Research Reviews* 47
(2018): 183–97; 61; Luigi Fontana, Jamil Nehme, and Marco Demaria,
"Caloric Restriction and Cellular Senescence," *Mechanisms of Ageing
and Development* 176 (2018): 19–23.

p. 71 . *Intermittent fasting suppresses this cellular activity*: in Young Choi,
Changhan Lee, and Valter D. Longo, "Nutrition and Fasting Mimicking
Diets in the Prevention and Treatment of Autoimmune Diseases and
Immunosenescence," *Molecular and Cellular Endocrinology* 455 (2017):
4–12.

p. 73   *Circadian rhythm and chronic pain*: Andrew E. Warfield, Jonathan F.
Prather, and William D. Todd, "Systems and Circuits Linking Chronic
Pain and Circadian Rhythms," *Frontiers in Neuroscience* 15 (2021): 829.

p. 73   *Early time-restricted eating*: Humaira Jamshed, Robbie A. Beyl,
Deborah L. Della Manna, Eddy S. Yang, Eric Ravussin, and Courtney
M. Peterson, "Early Time-Restricted Feeding Improves 24-Hour Glucose Levels and Affects Markers of the Circadian Clock, Aging,
and Autophagy in Humans," *Nutrients* 11, no. 6 (2019): 1234.

p. 74   *Adopting a low-carbohydrate diet...resulted in less pain*: Larissa J.

Strath, Catherine D. Jones, Alan Philip George, Shannon L. Lukens, Shannon A. Morrison, Taraneh Soleymani, Julie L. Locher, Barbara A. Gower, and Robert E. Sorge, "The Effect of Low-Carbohydrate and Low-Fat Diets on Pain in Individuals with Knee Osteoarthritis," *Pain Medicine* 21, no. 1 (2020): 150–60.

p. 74　*A Mediterranean-style diet*: Casuarina Forsyth, Matina Kouvari, Nathan M. D'Cunha, Ekavi N. Georgousopoulou, Demosthenes B. Panagiotakos, Duane D. Mellor, Jane Kellett, and Nenad Naumovski, "The Effects of the Mediterranean Diet on Rheumatoid Arthritis Prevention and Treatment: A Systematic Review of Human Prospective Studies," *Rheumatology International* 38, no. 5 (2018): 737–47.

Chapter 4: Revitalize

p. 83　*Movement offers us pleasure*: Kelly McGonigal, *The Joy of Movement: How Exercise Helps Us Find Happiness, Hope, Connection, and Courage* (New York: Avery, 2019).

p. 84　*People who exercised regularly had less chronic musculoskeletal pain*: Helene Sulutvedt Holth, Hanne Kine Buchardt Werpen, John-Anker Zwart, and Knut Hagen, "Physical Inactivity Is Associated with Chronic Musculoskeletal Complaints 11 Years Later: Results from the Nord-Trøndelag Health Study," *BMC Musculoskeletal Disorders* 9, no. 1 (2008): 1–7.

p. 84　*The more physically inactive a person is*: Andrew J. Teichtahl, Donna M. Urquhart, Yuanyuan Wang, Anita E. Wluka, Richard O'Sullivan, Graeme Jones, and Flavia M. Cicuttini, "Physical Inactivity Is Associated with Narrower Lumbar Intervertebral Discs, High Fat Content of Paraspinal Muscles and Low Back Pain and Disability," *Arthritis Research and Therapy* 17, no. 1 (2015): 1–7.

p. 84　*Prolonged sitting is associated with biochemical markers*: Thomas Yates, Kamlesh Khunti, Emma G. Wilmot, Emer Brady, David Webb, Bala Srinivasan, Joe Henson, Duncan Talbot, and Melanie J. Davies, "Self-Reported Sitting Time and Markers of Inflammation, Insulin Resistance, and Adiposity," *American Journal of Preventive Medicine* 42, no. 1 (2012): 1–7.

p. 84　*More time spent sitting correlated with higher rates of inflammatory diseases*: Teruhide Koyama, Nagato Kuriyama, Etsuko Ozaki, Satomi

Tomida, Ritei Uehara, Yuichiro Nishida, Chisato Shimanoe, et al., "Sedentary Time Is Associated with Cardiometabolic Diseases in a Large Japanese Population: A Cross-Sectional Study," *Journal of Athero-sclerosis and Thrombosis* 27, no. 10 (2020): 1097–1107.

p. 85   *A greater risk of dying from cancer*: Susan C. Gilchrist, Virginia J. Howard, Tomi Akinyemiju, Suzanne E. Judd, Mary Cushman, Steven P. Hooker, and Keith M. Diaz, "Association of Sedentary Behavior with Cancer Mortality in Middle-Aged and Older US Adults," *JAMA Oncology* 6, no. 8 (2020): 1210–17.

p. 85   Neuroprotective, *meaning that it protects the brain*: Cristy Phillips and Atoossa Fahimi, "Immune and Neuroprotective Effects of Physical Activity on the Brain in Depression," *Frontiers in Neuroscience* 12 (2018): 498.

p. 85   *Exercise itself can reduce chronic pain*: David Rice, Jo Nijs, Eva Kosek, Timothy Wideman, Monika I. Hasenbring, Kelli Koltyn, Thomas Graven-Nielsen, and Andrea Polli, "Exercise-Induced Hypoalgesia in Pain-Free and Chronic Pain Populations: State of the Art and Future Directions," *Journal of Pain* 20, no. 11 (2019): 1249–66.

p. 86   *Exercise increases pain tolerance*: Daniel L. Belavy, Jessica Van Oosterwijck, Matthew Clarkson, Evy Dhondt, Niamh L. Mundell, Clint T. Miller, and Patrick J. Owen, "Pain Sensitivity Is Reduced by Exercise Training: Evidence from a Systematic Review and Meta-analysis," *Neuroscience and Biobehavioral Reviews* 120 (2021): 100–108.

p. 87   *safer, better alternatives to narcotics*: Allan H. Goldfarb, Robert R. Kraemer, and Brandon A. Baiamonte, "Endogenous Opiates and Exercise-Related Hypoalgesia," in *Endocrinology of Physical Activity and Sport.*, ed. A. Hackney and N. Constantini (New York: Springer, 2020), 19–39.

p. 87   *medications called* exercise mimetics: Davide Guerrieri, Hyo Youl Moon, and Henriette van Praag, "Exercise in a Pill: The Latest on Exercise Mimetics," *Brain Plasticity* 2, no. 2 (2017): 153–69.

p. 87   *Moderate-intensity exercise decreases pain*: Kelly M. Naugle, Keith E. Naugle, Roger B. Fillingim, Brian Samuels, and Joseph L. Riley III, "Intensity Thresholds for Aerobic Exercise–Induced Hypoalgesia," *Medicine and Science in Sports and Exercise* 46, no. 4 (2014): 817.

p. 87   *Leg exercises can decrease shoulder pain*: Craig A. Wassinger, Logan Lumpkins, and Gisela Sole, "Lower Extremity Aerobic Exercise as a Treatment for Shoulder Pain," *International Journal of Sports Physical Therapy* 15, no. 1 (2020): 74.

p. 87   *Medical marijuana (cannabis) has been shown*: Bjorn Jensen, Jeffrey
         Chen, Tim Furnish, and Mark Wallace, "Medical Marijuana and
         Chronic Pain: A Review of Basic Science and Clinical Evidence," *Cur-
         rent Pain and Headache Reports* 19, no. 10 (2015): 1–9.

p. 88   *Moderately intense activity...activates the production of endocannabi-
         noids*: P.B. Sparling, A. Giuffrida, D. Piomelli, L. Rosskopf, and A.
         Dietrich, "Exercise Activates the Endocannabinoid System," *Neurore-
         port* 14, no. 17 (2003): 2209–11.

p. 88   *Exercise increases levels of serotonin*: Lucas V. Lima, Thiago S.S. Abner,
         and Kathleen A. Sluka, "Does Exercise Increase or Decrease Pain?
         Central Mechanisms Underlying These Two Phenomena," *Journal of
         Physiology* 595, no. 13 (2017): 4141–50.

p. 88   *Myokines help prevent muscle wasting*: Marta Gomarasca, Giuseppe
         Banfi, and Giovanni Lombardi, "Myokines: The Endocrine Coupling of
         Skeletal Muscle and Bone," *Advances in Clinical Chemistry* 94 (2020):
         155–218.

p. 88   *Exercise as an anti-inflammatory treatment*: Fabiana B. Benatti and
         Bente K. Pedersen, "Exercise as an Anti-Inflammatory Therapy for
         Rheumatic Diseases: Myokine Regulation," *Nature Reviews Rheumatol-
         ogy* 11, no. 2 (2015): 86–97.

p. 88   *Moderate-intensity walking resulted in less inflammation*: Yunsuk Koh
         and Kyung-Shin Park, "Responses of Inflammatory Cytokines Fol-
         lowing Moderate Intensity Walking Exercise in Overweight or Obese
         Individuals," *Journal of Exercise Rehabilitation* 13, no. 4 (2017): 472.

p. 88   *Twenty minutes of moderate walking lowered inflammation*: Stoyan
         Dimitrov, Elaine Hulteng, and Suzi Hong, "Inflammation and Exercise:
         Inhibition of Monocytic Intracellular TNF Production by Acute Exer-
         cise Via B2-Adrenergic Activation," *Brain, Behavior, and Immunity* 61
         (2017): 60–68.

p. 90   *Lifespan increased in women*: I-Min Lee, Eric J. Shiroma, Masamitsu
         Kamada, David R. Bassett, Charles E. Matthews, and Julie E. Buring,
         "Association of Step Volume and Intensity with All-Cause Mortality in
         Older Women," *JAMA Internal Medicine* 179, no. 8 (2019): 1105–12.

p. 91   *Using a smartphone*: Wouter M.A. Franssen, Gregor H.L.M. Franssen,
         Jan Spaas, Francesca Solmi, and Bert O. Eijnde, "Can Consumer Wear-
         able Activity Tracker-Based Interventions Improve Physical Activity
         and Cardiometabolic Health in Patients with Chronic Diseases? A

Systematic Review and Meta-analysis of Randomised Controlled Trials," *International Journal of Behavioral Nutrition and Physical Activity* 17 (2020): 1–20.

p. 92   *Medium-tempo music improved enjoyment:* Costas I. Karageorghis, Leighton Jones, Luke W. Howard, Rhys M. Thomas, Panayiotis Moulashis, and Sam J. Santich, "When It Hiits, You Feel No Pain: Psychological and Psychophysiological Effects of Respite-Active Music in High-Intensity Interval Training," *Journal of Sport and Exercise Psychology* 43, no. 1 (2021): 41–52.

p. 94   *A free manual on proper material handling:* Centers for Disease Control and Prevention, National Institute for Occupational Safety and Health, *Ergonomic Guidelines for Manual Material Handling,* April 2007, www.cdc.gov/niosh/docs/2007-131/default.html.

p. 98   *HIIT reduces inflammation:* Ljiljana Plavsic, Olivera M. Knezevic, Aleksandar Sovtic, Predrag Minic, Rade Vukovic, Ilijana Mazibrada, Olivera Stanojlovic, Dragan Hrncic, Aleksandra Rasic-Markovic, and Djuro Macut, "Effects of High-Intensity Interval Training and Nutrition Advice on Cardiometabolic Markers and Aerobic Fitness in Adolescent Girls with Obesity," *Applied Physiology, Nutrition, and Metabolism* 45, no. 3 (2020): 294–300.

p. 98   *A study of older adults with rheumatoid arthritis:* David B. Bartlett, Leslie H. Willis, Cris A. Slentz, Andrew Hoselton, Leslie Kelly, Janet L. Huebner, Virginia B. Kraus, et al., "Ten Weeks of High-Intensity Interval-Walk Training Is Associated with Reduced Disease Activity and Improved Innate Immune Function in Older Adults with Rheumatoid Arthritis: A Pilot Study," *Arthritis Research and Therapy* 20, no. 1 (2018): 1–15.

p. 98   *Studies involving HIIT and chronic low back pain:* Jonas Verbrugghe, Anouk Agten, Sjoerd Stevens, Dominique Hansen, Christophe Demoulin, Bert O. Eijnde, Frank Vandenabeele, and Annick Timmermans, "High Intensity Training to Treat Chronic Nonspecific Low Back Pain: Effectiveness of Various Exercise Modes," *Journal of Clinical Medicine* 9, no. 8 (2020): 2401.

p. 98   *Outdoor exercise resulted in less tension:* Jo Thompson Coon, Kate Boddy, Ken Stein, Rebecca Whear, Joanne Barton, and Michael H. Depledge, "Does Participating in Physical Activity in Outdoor Natural Environments Have a Greater Effect on Physical and Mental Wellbeing

Than Physical Activity Indoors? A Systematic Review," *Environmental Science and Technology* 45, no. 5 (2011): 1761–72.

p. 99   *Forest bathing reduces physical, mental, and emotional stress*: Yuko Tsunetsugu, Bum-Jin Park, Juyoung Lee, Takahide Kagawa, and Yoshifumi Miyazaki, "Psychological Relaxation Effect of Forest Therapy: Results of Field Experiments in 19 Forests in Japan Involving 228 Participants," *Nihon eiseigaku zasshi (Japanese Journal of Hygiene)* 66, no. 4 (2011): 670–76; 30; Bum Jin Park, Yuko Tsunetsugu, Tamami Kasetani, Takahide Kagawa, and Yoshifumi Miyazaki, "The Physiological Effects of Shinrin-Yoku (Taking in the Forest Atmosphere or Forest Bathing): Evidence from Field Experiments in 24 Forests Across Japan," *Environmental Health and Preventive Medicine* 15, no. 1 (2010): 18–26.

Chapter 5: Recharge

p. 103   *Sleep that knits up the raveled sleave*: William Shakespeare, *MacBeth*. (London: Macmillian Collector's Library, 2016), act II, scene 2.

p. 104   *Sleep deprivation can result in greater impairment*: Joanna Lowrie and Helen Brownlow, "The Impact of Sleep Deprivation and Alcohol on Driving: A Comparative Study," *BMC Public Health* 20, no. 1 (2020): 1–9.

p. 104   *People with poor sleep quality have more cortical atrophy*: Claire E. Sexton, Andreas B. Storsve, Kristine B. Walhovd, Heidi Johansen-Berg, and Anders M. Fjell, "Poor Sleep Quality Is Associated with Increased Cortical Atrophy in Community-Dwelling Adults," *Neurology* 83, no. 11 (2014): 967–73.

p. 104   *Insufficient sleep decreases resilience*: S. Hakki Onen, Abdelkrim Alloui, Annette Gross, Alain Eschallier, and Claude Dubray, "The Effects of Total Sleep Deprivation, Selective Sleep Interruption and Sleep Recovery on Pain Tolerance Thresholds in Healthy Subjects," *Journal of Sleep Research* 10, no. 1 (2001): 35–42.

p. 105   *Shorter sleep durations…are correlated with higher levels of inflammation*: Martica H. Hall, Stephen F. Smagula, Robert M. Boudreau, Hilsa N. Ayonayon, Suzanne E. Goldman, Tamara B. Harris, Barbara L. Naydeck, et al., "Association between Sleep Duration and Mortality Is Mediated by Markers of Inflammation and Health in Older Adults: The Health, Aging and Body Composition Study," *Sleep* 38, no. 2 (2015): 189–95.

p. 105   *Shorter sleep duration is also associated with obesity*: Gregor Hasler,

Daniel J. Buysse, Richard Klaghofer, Alex Gamma, Vladeta Ajdacic, Dominique Eich, Wulf Rössler, and Jules Angst, "The Association between Short Sleep Duration and Obesity in Young Adults: A 13-Year Prospective Study," *Sleep* 27, no. 4 (2004): 661–66.

p. 105   *Insufficient deep sleep*: Eileen B. Leary, Kathleen T. Watson, Sonia Ancoli-Israel, Susan Redline, Kristine Yaffe, Laurel A. Ravelo, Paul E. Peppard, et al., "Association of Rapid Eye Movement Sleep with Mortality in Middle-Aged and Older Adults," *JAMA Neurology* 77, no. 10 (2020): 1241–51.

p. 105   *A study of people sent to pain physicians*: Issy Pilowsky, I. Crettenden, and M. Townley, "Sleep Disturbance in Pain Clinic Patients," *Pain* 23, no. 1 (1985): 27–33.

p. 105   *Poor sleep is also documented among people with rheumatoid arthritis*: Lynette A. Menefee, Mitchell J. M. Cohen, Whitney R. Anderson, Karl Doghramji, Evan D. Frank, and Hochang Lee, "Sleep Disturbance and Nonmalignant Chronic Pain: A Comprehensive Review of the Literature," *Pain Medicine* 1, no. 2 (2000): 156–72.

p. 106   *Sleeping for five hours or less per night*: Min Young Chun, Bum-Joo Cho, Sang Ho Yoo, Bumjo Oh, Ju-Seop Kang, and Cholog Yeon, "Association between Sleep Duration and Musculoskeletal Pain: The Korea National Health and Nutrition Examination Survey 2010–2015," *Medicine* 97, no. 50 (2018).

p. 106   *People who slept less for ten consecutive nights*: Monika Haack, Elsa Sanchez, and Janet M. Mullington, "Elevated Inflammatory Markers in Response to Prolonged Sleep Restriction Are Associated with Increased Pain Experience in Healthy Volunteers," *Sleep* 30, no. 9 (2007): 1145–52.

p. 106   *Catching up on sleep after nights of disrupted sleep*: Onen, Alloui, Gross, et al., "The Effects of Total Sleep Deprivation."

p. 106   *A more diverse, healthy gut microbiome correlates with better sleep*: Robert P. Smith, Cole Easson, Sarah M. Lyle, Ritishka Kapoor, Chase P. Donnelly, Eileen J. Davidson, Esha Parikh, Jose V. Lopez, and Jaime L. Tartar, "Gut Microbiome Diversity Is Associated with Sleep Physiology in Humans," *PLoS One* 14, no. 10 (2019): e0222394.

p. 108   *Correlation between poor sleep and higher body weight*: Shahrad Taheri, Ling Lin, Diane Austin, Terry Young, and Emmanuel Mignot, "Short

Sleep Duration Is Associated with Reduced Leptin, Elevated Ghrelin, and Increased Body Mass Index," *PLoS Medicine* 1, no. 3 (2004): e62.

p. 108　*People who slept less during the week*: Christopher M. Depner, Edward L. Melanson, Robert H. Eckel, Janet K. Snell-Bergeon, Leigh Perreault, Bryan C. Bergman, Janine A. Higgins, et al., "Ad Libitum Weekend Recovery Sleep Fails to Prevent Metabolic Dysregulation During a Repeating Pattern of Insufficient Sleep and Weekend Recovery Sleep," *Current Biology* 29, no. 6 (2019): 957–67.

p. 109　*CBT-I has been found to lengthen sleep time*: Kyla Petrie and Elizabeth Matzkin, "Can Pharmacological and Non-Pharmacological Sleep Aids Reduce Post-Operative Pain and Opioid Usage? A Review of the Literature," *Orthopedic Reviews* 11, no. 4 (2019): 8306.

p. 110　*Eating near bedtime results in higher calorie consumption*: Kathryn J. Reid, Kelly G. Baron, and Phyllis C. Zee, "Meal Timing Influences Daily Caloric Intake in Healthy Adults," *Nutrition Research* 34, no. 11 (2014): 930–35.

p. 112　*People who wore amber lenses two hours before bedtime*: Ari Shechter, Elijah Wookhyun Kim, Marie-Pierre St-Onge, and Andrew J. Westwood, "Blocking Nocturnal Blue Light for Insomnia: A Randomized Controlled Trial," *Journal of Psychiatric Research* 96 (2018): 196–202.

p. 113　*Being grateful at bedtime*: Alex M. Wood, Stephen Joseph, Joanna Lloyd, and Samuel Atkins, "Gratitude Influences Sleep Through the Mechanism of Pre-Sleep Cognitions," *Journal of Psychosomatic Research* 66, no. 1 (2009): 43–48.

p. 113　*Bedtime mindfulness and meditation practices*: David S. Black, Gillian A. O'Reilly, Richard Olmstead, Elizabeth C. Breen, and Michael R. Irwin, "Mindfulness Meditation and Improvement in Sleep Quality and Daytime Impairment among Older Adults with Sleep Disturbances: A Randomized Clinical Trial," *JAMA Internal Medicine* 175, no. 4 (2015): 494–501.

Chapter 6: Refresh

p. 121　*During my own years of chronic pain*: Martha Beck, *The Way of Integrity: Finding the Path to Your True Self* (New York: Viking, 2021), 89.

p. 122　*Suffering translates to a negative distortion*: Auro del Giglio, "Suffering-

Based Medicine: Practicing Scientific Medicine with a Humanistic Approach," *Medicine, Health Care and Philosophy* 23, no. 2 (2020): 215–19.

p. 125 *The number one cause of their low back pain was stress*: "Perceived Causes of Back Pain among U.S. Adults as of 2017," Statista, September 3, 2019, www.statista.com/statistics/680812/self-reported-causes-of -back-pain-adults-us.

p. 125 *Psychosocial stress ... results in weight gain and elevated markers of inflammation*: Jason P. Block, Yulei He, Alan M. Zaslavsky, Lin Ding, and John Z. Ayanian, "Psychosocial Stress and Change in Weight among US Adults," *American Journal of Epidemiology* 170, no. 2 (2009): 181–92; Andrew H. Miller, Vladimir Maletic, and Charles L. Raison, "Inflammation and Its Discontents: The Role of Cytokines in the Pathophysiology of Major Depression," *Biological Psychiatry* 65, no. 9 (2009): 732–41.

p. 125 *When healthy people were placed under acute psychosocial stress*: Michel Mertens, Linda Hermans, Jessica Van Oosterwijck, Lotte Meert, Geert Crombez, Filip Struyf, and Mira Meeus, "The Result of Acute Induced Psychosocial Stress on Pain Sensitivity and Modulation in Healthy People," *Pain Physician* 23, no. 6 (2020): E703–E712.

p. 126 *Insufficient sleep increases cortisol*: Mathieu Nollet, William Wisden, and Nicholas P. Franks, "Sleep Deprivation and Stress: A Reciprocal Relationship," *Interface Focus* 10, no. 3 (2020): 20190092.

p. 126 *During stressful times*: Norman Pecoraro, Faith Reyes, Francisca Gomez, Aditi Bhargava, and Mary F. Dallman, "Chronic Stress Promotes Palatable Feeding, Which Reduces Signs of Stress: Feedforward and Feedback Effects of Chronic Stress," *Endocrinology* 145, no. 8 (2004): 3754–62.

p. 126 *Chronic stress also changes our gut microbiome*: Ryan Rieder, Paul J. Wisniewski, Brandon L. Alderman, and Sara C. Campbell, "Microbes and Mental Health: A Review," *Brain, Behavior, and Immunity* 66 (2017): 9–17.

p. 126 *Stress, smoking, obesity, lack of movement, and an unhealthy diet accelerate telomere damage*: Masood A. Shammas, "Telomeres, Lifestyle, Cancer, and Aging," *Current Opinion in Clinical Nutrition and Metabolic Care* 14, no. 1 (2011): 28.

p. 127 *Mindfulness meditation may increase telomere length*: Nicola S. Schutte and John M. Malouff, "A Meta-Analytic Review of the Effects of Mindfulness Meditation on Telomerase Activity," *Psychoneuroendocrinology* 42 (2014): 45–48.

p. 130   *Meditation decreased levels of the inflammatory markers*: Lara Hilton, Susanne Hempel, Brett A. Ewing, Eric Apaydin, Lea Xenakis, Sydne Newberry, Ben Colaiaco, et al., "Mindfulness Meditation for Chronic Pain: Systematic Review and Meta-analysis," *Annals of Behavioral Medicine* 51, no. 2 (2017): 199–213.

p. 130   *A study of US marines*: Johnson, Douglas C. Johnson, Nathaniel J. Thom, Elizabeth A. Stanley, Lori Haase, Alan N. Simmons, Pei-an B. Shih, Wesley K. Thompson, Eric G. Potterat, Thomas R. Minor, and Martin P. Paulus, "Modifying Resilience Mechanisms in At-Risk Individuals: A Controlled Study of Mindfulness Training in Marines Preparing for Deployment," *American Journal of Psychiatry* 171, no. 8 (2014): 844–53.

p. 130   *Mindfulness and meditation techniques decrease low back pain*: Linda E. Carlson, "Mindfulness-Based Interventions for Physical Conditions: A Narrative Review Evaluating Levels of Evidence," *ISRN Psychiatry* 2012 (November 2012): 651583.

p. 130   *The part of the brain involved in learning*: Britta K. Hölzel, James Carmody, Mark Vangel, Christina Congleton, Sita M. Yerramsetti, Tim Gard, and Sara W. Lazar, "Mindfulness Practice Leads to Increases in Regional Brain Gray Matter Density," *Psychiatry Research: Neuroimaging* 191, no. 1 (2011): 36–43; Bolton K. H. Chau, Kati Keuper, Mandy Lo, Kwok-Fai So, Chetwyn C. H. Chan, and Tatia M. C. Lee, "Meditation-Induced Neuroplastic Changes of the Prefrontal Network Are Associated with Reduced Valence Perception in Older People," *Brain and Neuroscience Advances* 2 (2018): 2398212818771822.

p. 130   *A study of adults with chronic low back pain*: Daniel C. Cherkin, Karen J. Sherman, Benjamin H. Balderson, Andrea J. Cook, Melissa L. Anderson, Rene J. Hawkes, Kelly E. Hansen, and Judith A. Turner, "Effect of Mindfulness-Based Stress Reduction Vs Cognitive Behavioral Therapy or Usual Care on Back Pain and Functional Limitations in Adults with Chronic Low Back Pain: a Randomized Clinical Trial," *JAMA* 315, no. 12 (2016): 1240–49.

p. 132   *More screen time correlates with obesity*: Thomas N. Robinson, Jorge A. Banda, Lauren Hale, Amy Shirong Lu, Frances Fleming-Milici, Sandra

L. Calvert, and Ellen Wartella, "Screen Media Exposure and Obesity in Children and Adolescents," *Pediatrics* 140, supp. 2 (2017): S97–S101.

p. 133 *Cell phone use and driving*: Jon Atwood, Feng Guo, Greg Fitch, and Thomas A. Dingus, "The Driver-Level Crash Risk Associated with Daily Cellphone Use and Cellphone Use While Driving," *Accident Analysis and Prevention* 119 (2018): 149–54.

p. 133 *Responding to multiple stimuli at the same time*: Mark A. Wetherell and Kirsty Carter, "The Multitasking Framework: The Effects of Increasing Workload on Acute Psychobiological Stress Reactivity," *Stress and Health* 30, no. 2 (2014): 103–9.

p. 136 *Meditation decreased knee pain*: Kim E. Innes, Terry Kit Selfe, Sahiti Kandati, Sijin Wen, and Zenzi Huysmans, "Effects of Mantra Meditation versus Music Listening on Knee Pain, Function, and Related Outcomes in Older Adults with Knee Osteoarthritis: an Exploratory Randomized Clinical Trial (RCT)," *Evidence-Based Complementary and Alternative Medicine* 2018 (August 2018): 7683897.

p. 138 *Tactical breathing*: Stefan Röttger, Dominique A. Theobald, Johanna Abendroth, and Thomas Jacobsen, "The Effectiveness of Combat Tactical Breathing as Compared with Prolonged Exhalation," *Applied Psychophysiology and Biofeedback* 46, no. 1 (2021): 19–28.

p. 140 *People who believe they are being punished or abandoned by God*: Kenneth I. Pargament, Harold G. Koenig, Nalini Tarakeshwar, and June Hahn, "Religious Struggle as a Predictor of Mortality among Medically Ill Elderly Patients: A 2-Year Longitudinal Study," *Archives of Internal Medicine* 161, no. 15 (2001): 1881–85.

p. 141 *"The experience of pain arises from both physiological and psychological factors"*: Tor D. Wager, James K. Rilling, Edward E. Smith, Alex Sokolik, Kenneth L. Casey, Richard J. Davidson, Stephen M. Kosslyn, Robert M. Rose, and Jonathan D. Cohen, "Placebo-Induced Changes in FMRI in the Anticipation and Experience of Pain," *Science* 303, no. 5661 (2004): 1162–67.

p. 141 *Better coping responses correlate with a quicker recovery*: John A. Sturgeon and Alex J. Zautra, "Resilience: A New Paradigm for Adaptation to Chronic Pain," *Current Pain and Headache Reports* 14, no. 2 (2010): 105–12.

p. 143 *It takes three positive thoughts or comments*: Barbara L. Fredrickson and Marcial F. Losada, "Positive Affect and the Complex Dynamics of Human Flourishing," *American Psychologist* 60, no. 7 (2005): 678.

p. 146   *78 percent of people who underwent a sham surgery*: Wayne B. Jonas, Cindy Crawford, Luana Colloca, Ted J. Kaptchuk, Bruce Moseley, Franklin G. Miller, Levente Kriston, Klaus Linde, and Karin Meissner, "To What Extent Are Surgery and Invasive Procedures Effective Beyond a Placebo Response? A Systematic Review with Meta-analysis of Randomised, Sham Controlled Trials," *BMJ Open* 5, no. 12 (2015): e009655.

p. 146   *The placebo effect triggers the release of natural painkillers*: Zev M. Medoff and Luana Colloca, "Placebo Analgesia: Understanding the Mechanisms," *Pain Management* 5, no. 2 (2015): 89–96; Beth D. Darnall and Luana Colloca, "Optimizing Placebo and Minimizing Nocebo to Reduce Pain, Catastrophizing, and Opioid Use: A Review of the Science and an Evidence-Informed Clinical Toolkit," *International Review of Neurobiology* 139 (2018): 129–57.

p. 147   *This outlook sets us up for failure*: Nicole Corsi and Luana Colloca, "Placebo and Nocebo Effects: The Advantage of Measuring Expectations and Psychological Factors," *Frontiers in Psychology* 8 (2017): 308.

p. 147   *Positive pain expectations activate opioid pain-relieving pathways*: Damien G. Finniss, Ted J. Kaptchuk, Franklin Miller, and Fabrizio Benedetti, "Biological, Clinical, and Ethical Advances of Placebo Effects," *Lancet* 375, no. 9715 (2010): 686–95; 31. Thompson, Kathryn A. Thompson, Hailey W. Bulls, Kimberly T. Sibille, Emily J. Bartley, Toni L. Glover, Ellen L. Terry, Ivana A. Vaughn, et al., "Optimism and Psychological Resilience Are Beneficially Associated with Measures of Clinical and Experimental Pain in Adults with or At Risk for Knee Osteoarthritis," *Clinical Journal of Pain* 34, no. 12 (2018): 1164; Emily J. Bartley, Shreela Palit, Roger B. Fillingim, and Michael E. Robinson, "Multisystem Resiliency as a Predictor of Physical and Psychological Functioning in Older Adults with Chronic Low Back Pain," *Frontiers in Psychology* 10 (2019): 1932.

p. 149   *People with a positive outlook recover from physical and psychological stressors*: Michele M. Tugade and Barbara L. Fredrickson, "Resilient Individuals Use Positive Emotions to Bounce Back from Negative Emotional Experiences," *Journal of Personality and Social Psychology* 86, no. 2 (2004): 320–33.

p. 154   *Patients who look at nature views*: Erin Largo-Wight, "Cultivating Healthy Places and Communities: Evidenced-Based Nature Contact

Recommendations," *International Journal of Environmental Health Research* 21, no. 1 (2011): 41–61.

p. 154   *Hospitalized patients with windows offering a view of nature*: Sara Malenbaum, Francis J. Keefe, Amanda Williams, Roger Ulrich, and Tamara J. Somers, "Pain in Its Environmental Context: Implications for Designing Environments to Enhance Pain Control," *Pain* 134, no. 3 (2008): 241–44.

Chapter 7: Relate

p. 163   *We need to more deeply appreciate*: Vivek H. Murthy, *Together: The Healing Power of Human Connection in a Sometimes Lonely World* (New York: Harper Wave, 2020).

p. 164   *Isolation or feeling lonely can be as deadly*: Julianne Holt-Lunstad, Timothy B. Smith, Mark Baker, Tyler Harris, and David Stephenson, "Loneliness and Social Isolation as Risk Factors for Mortality: A Meta-Analytic Review," *Perspectives on Psychological Science* 10, no. 2 (2015): 227–37.

p. 164   *It chips away at our health and pain tolerance*: John T. Cacioppo and Stephanie Cacioppo, "Social Relationships and Health: The Toxic Effects of Perceived Social Isolation," *Social and Personality Psychology Compass* 8, no. 2 (2014): 58–72.

p. 164   *Solitary confinement correlates with more depression*: Keramet Reiter, Joseph Ventura, David Lovell, Dallas Augustine, Melissa Barragan, Thomas Blair, Kelsie Chesnut, et al., "Psychological Distress in Solitary Confinement: Symptoms, Severity, and Prevalence in the United States, 2017–2018," *American Journal of Public Health* 110, supp. 1 (2020): S56–S62.

p. 164   *Those in solitary confinement had more orthopaedic pain*: Justin D. Strong, Keramet Reiter, Gabriela Gonzalez, Rebecca Tublitz, Dallas Augustine, Melissa Barragan, Kelsie Chesnut, Pasha Dashtgard, Natalie Pifer, and Thomas R. Blair, "The Body in Isolation: The Physical Health Impacts of Incarceration in Solitary Confinement," *PloS One* 15, no. 10 (2020): e0238510.

p. 164   *Only three weeks into stay-at-home orders*: William D. S. Killgore, Sara A. Cloonan, Emily C. Taylor, and Natalie S. Dailey, "Loneliness: A Signature Mental Health Concern in the Era of COVID-19," *Psychiatry Research* 290 (2020): 113117.

p. 165   *Resilience greater in those who felt more socially supported*: William D. S. Killgore, Emily C. Taylor, Sara A. Cloonan, and Natalie S. Dailey, "Psychological Resilience during the COVID-19 Lockdown," *Psychiatry Research* 291 (2020): 113216.

p. 165   *Lonely people are more likely to develop difficulties*: Carla M. Perissinotto, Irena Stijacic Cenzer, and Kenneth E. Covinsky, "Loneliness in Older Persons: A Predictor of Functional Decline and Death," *Archives of Internal Medicine* 172, no. 14 (2012): 1078–84.

p. 165   *Poor social support could be used as a predictor*: Gabriele Buruck, Anne Tomaschek, Johannes Wendsche, Elke Ochsmann, and Denise Dörfel, "Psychosocial Areas of Worklife and Chronic Low Back Pain: A Systematic Review and Meta-analysis," *BMC Musculoskeletal Disorders* 20, no. 1 (2019): 1–16.

p. 165   *Social isolation results in weight gain*: Kassandra I. Alcaraz, Katherine S. Eddens, Jennifer L. Blase, W. Ryan Diver, Alpa V. Patel, Lauren R. Teras, Victoria L. Stevens, Eric J. Jacobs, and Susan M. Gapstur, "Social Isolation and Mortality in US Black and White Men and Women," *American Journal of Epidemiology* 188, no. 1 (2019): 102–9; Nonogaki Katsunori, Kana Nozue, and Yoshitomo Oka, "Social Isolation Affects the Development of Obesity and Type 2 Diabetes in Mice," *Endocrinology* 148, no. 10 (2007): 4658–66.

p. 166   *Good social relationships correlate with lower inflammatory markers*: Jodi Ford, Cindy Anderson, Shannon Gillespie, Carmen Giurgescu, Timiya Nolan, Alexandra Nowak, and Karen Patricia Williams, "Social Integration and Quality of Social Relationships as Protective Factors for Inflammation in a Nationally Representative Sample of Black Women," *Journal of Urban Health* 96, no. 1 (2019): 35–43; Eric B. Loucks, Lisa M. Sullivan, Ralph B. D'Agostino Sr, Martin G. Larson, Lisa F. Berkman, and Emelia J. Benjamin, "Social Networks and Inflammatory Markers in the Framingham Heart Study," *Journal of Biosocial Science* 38, no. 6 (2006): 835–42.

p. 166   *Social support and integration correlated with lower inflammation levels*: Bert N. Uchino, Ryan Trettevik, Robert G. Kent de Grey, Sierra Cronan, Jasara Hogan, and Brian R. W. Baucom, "Social Support, Social Integration, and Inflammatory Cytokines: A Meta-analysis," *Health Psychology* 37, no. 5 (2018): 462.

p. 167   *A person's risk of becoming obese increased*: Nicholas A. Christakis and James H. Fowler, "The Spread of Obesity in a Large Social Network

Over 32 Years," *New England Journal of Medicine* 357, no. 4 (2007): 370–79.

p. 167   *A spouse quitting smoking lowered the other person's likelihood of smoking*: Nicholas A. Christakis and James H. Fowler, "The Collective Dynamics of Smoking in a Large Social Network," *New England Journal of Medicine* 358, no. 21 (2008): 2249–58.

p. 168   *People surrounded by happy people are more likely to be happy*: James H. Fowler and Nicholas A. Christakis, "Dynamic Spread of Happiness in a Large Social Network: Longitudinal Analysis Over 20 Years in the Framingham Heart Study," *BMJ* (2008): 337:a2338.

p. 172   *"A state of complete physical, mental and social well-being"*: World Health Organization, "Constitution," www.who.int/about/governance /constitution.

p. 172   *The Centers for Disease Control and Prevention (CDC) elaborates the definition of well-being*: Centers for Disease Control and Prevention, "Health-Related Quality of Life, Well-Being Concepts," www.cdc.gov /hrqol/wellbeing.htm.

p. 173   *Higher levels of well-being are cultivated*: Sonja Lyubomirsky, *The Myths of Happiness: What Should Make You Happy but Doesn't, What Shouldn't Make You Happy but Does* (New York: Penguin, 2013).

p. 175   *One four-week study compared the well-being of people*: S. Katherine Nelson, Kristin Layous, Steven W. Cole, and Sonja Lyubomirsky, "Do Unto Others or Treat Yourself? The Effects of Prosocial and Self-Focused Behavior on Psychological Flourishing," *Emotion* 16, no. 6 (2016): 850.

p. 177   *Two groups of people who walked outside daily*: Virginia E. Sturm, Samir Datta, Ashlin R. K. Roy, Isabel J. Sible, Eena L. Kosik, Christina R. Veziris, Tiffany E. Chow, et al., "Big Smile, Small Self: Awe Walks Promote Prosocial Positive Emotions in Older Adults," *Emotion* (2020).

p. 177   *another microboost, gratitude, improves well-being*: Randy A. Sansone and Lori A. Sansone, "Gratitude and Well Being: The Benefits of Appreciation," *Psychiatry (Edgmont)* 7, no. 11 (2010): 18.

Chapter 8: The Path

p. 185   *It's impossible to predict the future*: Bill Burnett and Dave Evans, *Designing Your Life: How to Build a Well-Lived, Joyful Life* (New York: Alfred A. Knopf, 2016), 26.

Index

Page references followed by an italicized *t.* indicate tables. Page references followed by an italicized *fig.* indicate illustrations or material contained in their captions.

About the Author

Saloni Sharma, MD, LAc, is double board-certified in pain management and rehabilitation medicine. She is the medical director and founder of the Orthopaedic Integrative Health Center at Rothman Orthopaedics in Philadelphia and has treated thousands of patients. As a nationally recognized pain expert, she serves as co-chair for pain management and spine rehabilitation for the American Academy of Physical Medicine and Rehabilitation and as a member of the national Opioid Task Force. She has directed national courses on opioid alternatives and regularly speaks and advocates for ways to manage pain without medication.

Dr. Sharma is a fellow of the Andrew Weil Center for Integrative Medicine and has studied functional medicine and lifestyle medicine. She completed her acupuncture training at Harvard Medical School. She has studied yoga and meditation at Parmarth Niketan in Rishikesh, India, and mindfulness at Thomas Jefferson University. Dr. Sharma completed Stanford University's inaugural physician well-being director course. She has spoken at Google about ways to burn bright and improve well-being.

Dr. Sharma is a clinical assistant professor of rehabilitation medicine at Thomas Jefferson University and has published numerous research articles and textbook chapters. Her teaching skills were recognized with the Dean's Award for Excellence in Education at Sidney Kimmel Medical College. She is a Main Line Top Doctor (selected by her peers). Dr. Sharma served as a chief resident at Thomas Jefferson University Hospital and as chief fellow at Penn State Hershey Medical Center. She lives near Philadelphia.

www.salonisharmamd.com
@salonisharmamd